This book is to be returned on or before
the last date stamped below.

Neurophysiology of the Vestibular System

Advances in Oto-Rhino-Laryngology

Vol. 41

Series Editor
C.R. Pfaltz, Basel

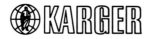

Basel · München · Paris · London · New York · New Delhi · Singapore · Tokyo · Sydney

Neurophysiology of the Vestibular System

Volume Editors
E. Pirodda, Bologna
O. Pompeiano, Pisa

95 figures, 2 color plates and 17 tables, 1988

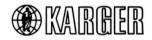

Basel · München · Paris · London · New York · New Delhi · Singapore · Tokyo · Sydney

Advances in Oto-Rhino-Laryngology

Library of Congress Cataloging-in-Publication Data
Bárány Society Meeting (1987: Bologna, Italy)
Neurophysiology of the vestibular system: selected
papers of the Bárány Society Meeting, Bologna,
June 1–4, 1987/volume editors, E. Pirodda, O. Pompeiano.
(Advances in oto-rhino-laryngology; vol. 41)
Includes bibliographies and index.
1. Vestibular apparatus–Physiology congresses. 2. Vestibular apparatus–Diseases–Congresses.
3. Neurophysiology–Congresses. I. Pirodda, Ettore, II. Pompeinao, O.
III. Title. IV. Series.
[DNLM: 1. Neurophysiology–congresses. 2. Vestibular Apparatus physiology–congresses.
3. Vestibular Function Tests–congresses. Wl AD701 v. 41/WV 255 B2255n 1987]
RF 16.A38 vol. 41 [QP471] 617'.51 s-dc19 [599'.0188] DNLM/DLC
ISBN 3–8055–4766–8

Bibliographic Indices
This publication is listed in bibliographic services, including Current Contents® and Index Medicus.

Drug Dosage
The authors and the publisher have exerted every effort to ensure that drug selection and dosage set forth in this text are in accord with current recommendations and practice at the time of publication. However, in view of ongoing research, changes in government regulations, and the constant flow of information relating to drug therapy and drug reactions, the reader is urged to check the package insert for each drug for any change in indications and dosage and for added warnings and precautions. This is particularly important when the recommended agent is a new and/or infrequently employed drug.

© Copyright 1988 by S. Karger AG, P.O. Box, CH–4009 Basel (Switzerland)
ISBN 3–8055–4766–8

Neurophysiology of the Vestibular System

This volume contains 44 selected papers presented at the Bárány Society Meeting, Bologna, July 1–4, 1987. 61 further papers are published as 'Clinical Testing of the Vestibular System', forming vol. 42 in the series Advances in Oto-Rhino-Laryngology (for contents see pp. VIII).

Contents

Contents

Contents

Clinical Testing of the Vestibular System

61 selected papers presented at the Bárány Society Meting, Bologna, June 1–4, 1987.
Published as vol. 42 in the series Advances in Oto-Rhino-Laryngology.

Contents

Contents

Contents   X

Adv. Oto-Rhino-Laryng., vol. 41, pp. 1–6 (Karger, Basel 1988)

Physiological Polarity of the Frog Utricle

Mamoru Suzuki, Yasuo Harada, Haruo Hirakawa, Katsuhiro Hirakawa, Ryo Omura, Akinori Kishimoto

Department of Otolaryngology, Hiroshima University, School of Medicine, Minamiku, Hiroshima, Japan

Introduction

The sensory cells of the otolithic organs are arranged in 2 opposite directions which form morphological polarity. However, physiological evidence of the polarity has not yet been fully demonstrated. This is probably due to difficulty in directly stimulating the otolithic organ. The authors attempted to confirm presence of physiological polarity on the frog utricular macula. A piece of a semicircular canal cupula was used to stimulate the macular sensory epithelia.

Materials and Methods

Six frogs (*Rana nigromaculata*) were used. After decapitation, the frogs' entire membranous labyrinths were removed and placed in Ringer's solution. The utricle and its nerve were isolated together with the anterior and the lateral semicircular canal ampullae from this preparation. Both the anterior and the posterior ampullary nerves were severed near the ampullae in order to allow recording of the nerve discharge solely from the utricle. A part of the lateral semicircular canal was inserted into a fine polyethylene tube in order to immobilize the entire preparation (fig. 1). Then, the utricular otoconia and the otoconial membrane were carefully removed by repeating a gentle flush and suction of the Ringer's solution.

The cupula of the anterior semicircular canal was removed from its ampulla. The cupula was sectioned in half, one of which was stuck into the tip of a glass microelectrode which was mounted on the micromanipulator. The base of the cupula was gently placed in

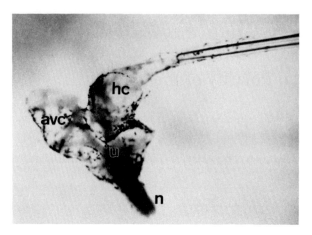

Fig. 1. Photograph of the preparation. avc = Anterior semicircular canal; hc = horizonal semicircular canal; u = utricle; n = nerve.

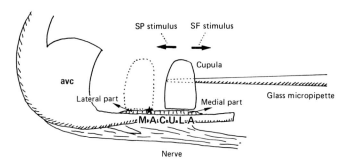

Fig. 2. A schema of the stimulation method. A halved cupula was stuck into the tip of the glass micropipette and the base of the cupula was placed on the macular surface. This allowed the cupular movement either toward the striola (SP stimulus) or away from the striola (SF stimulus).

the center of either the medial or the lateral part of the macula by controlling the micromanipulator. The micromanipulator allowed a sliding motion of the cupula on the macula by 1-μm steps (fig. 2). Cupula movement toward the striola was designated striolapetal (SP) movement, while movement away from the striola striolafugal (SF) movement (fig. 3). The utricular nerve compound action potential was recorded via a glass suction electrode. The duration of the stimulus was 10 s.

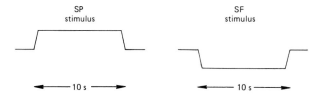

Fig. 3. Diagram of the stimulus. Both SP and SF stimuli lasted for 10 s with a short rise and fall time.

Results

When the medial part of the macula was stimulated, 5 μm of SP cupular movement elicited excitatory nerve discharge. The action potential tended to increase as the stimulus increased from 5 to 50 μm (fig. 4). Figure 5 compares the spike density histograms of the action potentials obtained from the SP stimuli to the medial (left column) and to the lateral (right column) parts of the macula. SP cupular movement resulted in stimulation of the action potentials, both in the medial and the lateral parts. SF stimulus did not evoke the action potential either in the medial or lateral parts.

Discussion

Physiology of the isolated frog semicircular canal had been intensively studied for many years. Yet only a few studies have been done on the peripheral physiology of the otolithic organs. This is probably because direct stimulation to the macula cannot be easily accomplished as compared to the semicircular canal. In this study the authors employed an isolated cupula to mechanically stimulate the macular sensory epithelia.

Our basic idea was that the cupula may well exert a displacement effect on the macula, since it serves as an optimum mechanotransducer of the semicircular canal. The present study proved that the cupula contributes to sensory cell excitation of the macula as well as of the crista. It was also observed that the excitatory responses always occurred from the cupula movement toward the striola, regardless of which part of the macula, medial or lateral, was stimulated. This confirms the presence of the physiological polarity, the direction of which is identical to the morphologically confirmed arrangement known as the morphological polarity.

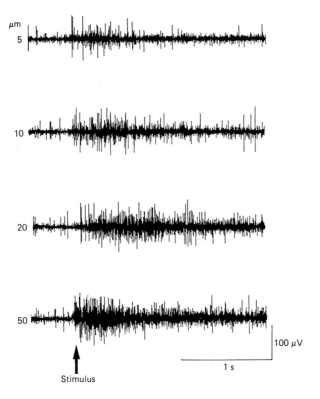

Fig. 4. The utricular nerve compound action potentials in response to the SP stimuli from 5 to 50 μm.

There are several studies which suggested that the physiological polarity exists. Loe et al. [3] recorded the activities of the cat utricular primary neuron under 360 degrees tilting stimulus. They showed that the maximum discharge was at the nose-up position, whereas the minimum discharge was at the 180° reversed position (nose-down position) thus suggesting that physiological polarity exists. Harada et al. [2] observed an on-off response from the frog utricular nerve by magnetically stimulating the macula, and indicated existence of a physiological polarity in the macula. In the present study the authors could establish directional excitability of the sensory cells by advocating more direct and quantitative stimulus to the macula.

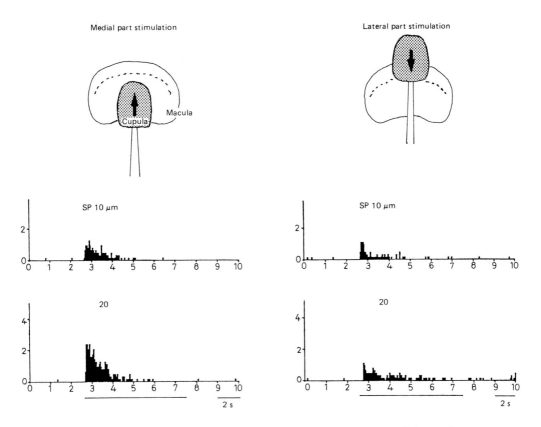

Fig. 5. The spike density histograms of the action potentials when the medial part of the macula (left column) and the lateral part of the macula (right column) are stimulated (SP stimulus). The action potentials were evoked from SP stimulus.

The otolithic primary neuron reportedly has physiological characteristics similar to the ampullary primary neuron in terms of regularity of the spontaneous discharge and the degree of adaptation. According to Fernandez et al. [1], the regular neurons tend not to adapt, while the irregular ones adapt more. Regarding the relationship between the regularity of the neuron and its gain, the regular neurons have smaller gain, while the irregular ones have larger gain. The same relationship between the regularity and the degree of adaptation was found in the frog posterior semicircular canal neurons. Physiological characteristics of the macular unit will be likewise elucidated using the technique advocated in this study.

References

1   Fernandez, C.; Goldberg, J.M.: Physiology of peripheral neurons innervating otolith organs of the squirrel monkey. I. Response to static tilts and to long-duration centrifugal force. J. Neurophysiol. *39:* 970–995 (1976).
2   Harada, Y.; Shirane, M.; Tagashira, N.; Suzuki, M.: Action potential of isolated frog utricle. Acta oto-lar. *406:* 143–148 (1984).
3   Loe, P.R.; Tomko, D.L.; Wertner, G.: The neural signal of angular head position in primary afferent vestibular nerve axons. J. Physiol. *230:* 29–50 (1973).

Mamoru Suzuki, MD, Department of Otolaryngology, Hiroshima University, School of Medicine, 1-2-3 Kasumi, Minamiku, Hiroshima 734 (Japan)

Adv. Oto-Rhino-Laryng., vol. 41, pp. 7–13 (Karger, Basel 1988)

Membrane Currents in Vestibular and Cochlear Hair Cells

Yasuo Harada, Yoshinori Sugata

Department of Otolaryngology, Hiroshima University, School of Medicine, Minamiku, Hiroshima, Japan

Introduction

The hair cell is a primary receptor of both the auditory and vestibular systems. Its function is mechanoelectrical transduction to the afferent neurons. It is known that a nerve impulse results from sodium inflow and potassium outflow through the neural membrane [3]. The similar transduction mechanism is proposed to be present in the hair cell. This study deals with the biophysical basis of the transduction mechanism of the single hair cell investigated by a whole cell clamp technique.

Materials and Method

Cell Preparation
Bullfrogs and guinea pigs were used. The sacculus and the cochlea were removed and were kept in Ca-free solution with papain (0.5 mg/ml) at room temperature for 30 min. After enzymatic treatment, the hair cells were dissociated into a single cell using a sharpened tungsten needle. The cell was placed in the culture dish which served as a recording chamber.

Recording
The composition of the external and the internal solutions are listed in table I. The capillary tubes with an outer diameter of 15 mm were used to fabricate a patch electrode. The electrodes were pulled on a horizontal type puller in two stages. The first pull thinned the capillary tube and the second pull thinned it to the point at which it separates into two electrodes with a diameter of about 1 μm. The electrodes were heat-polished by the platinum filament to create a smooth tip.

A culture dish was placed on the stage of an inverted microscope. The ground was taken through an Ag-AgCl wire electrode which was inserted into an agar-filled glass tube.

Table I. Composition of the solutions

	Na	K	Ca	TEA	Glucose
External solution					
Na sol.	113.5	5.4	3.0		10.0
Ca sol.	70.0	5.4	20.0	30.0	10.0

	K	Cs	EGTA	HEPES
Internal solution				
K sol.	130.0		5.0	10.0
Cs sol.		130.0	5.0	10.0

The recording electrode was connected to the probe of a patch clamp system EPC-7 through an Ag-AgCl wire. The pipette holder was fixed to the stage of a three-dimensional hydraulic manipulator. The electrode was gently pressed onto the cell membrane to obtain a gigaseal at the contact area (so-called 'patch'). Slight suction was applied to the electrode to rupture the patch of the membrane. After the patch was ruptured, the voltage or current clamp was proceeded.

Results

When the electrode was put into the external solution in the recording chamber, the electrode potential was equalized to the chamber potential. After rupture of the patch, the electrode potential became equal to the cell membrane potential. Therefore, the resting potential could be easily determined by maintaining the membrane current at zero, since no membrane current takes place at the resting potential. The resting potentials of the hair cells measured were from −40 to −75 mV.

Whole Cell Recording under the Voltage Clamp

After forming a gigaseal the patch was ruptured by additional suction. Electrical contact with the inside of the cell was indicated by a sudden increase in the capacitive transients from the level of the test pulse and a shift of the current level (fig. 1).

When depolarizing voltage pulses were applied to the cells at the holding potential, biphasic membrane currents consisting of the initial inward current and the following outward current were obtained in Na solution

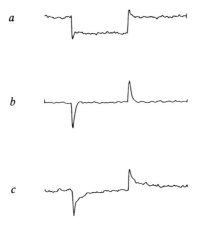

Fig. 1. Electrode currents. *a* Electrode current when electrode is in external solution. *b* Gigaseal is formed. Electrode current is almost zero. *c* Electrode current after rupture of the patch.

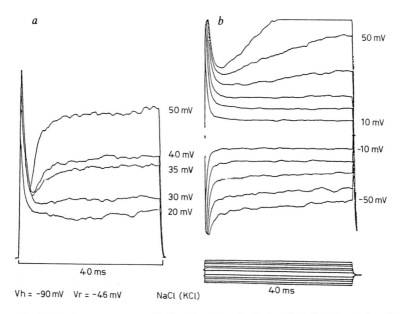

Fig. 2. Membrane currents of hair cell. *a* Saccular hair cell. *b* Cochlear hair cell.

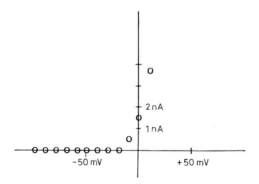

Fig. 3. Current-voltage relationship for the cochlear outer hair cell. The current was measured 40 ms after the start of a voltage step.

(fig. 2). In the vestibular hair cells, the outward currents were smaller than those of the cochlear hair cells.

When positive and negative voltage pulses were applied to the outer hair cell at a holding potential of −50 mV, a large outward current was found at the end of the voltage pulse (fig. 2). Membrane currents 40 ms after the start of the voltage pulse were corrected by subtracting the leakage current. The current-voltage relationship for this outer hair cell was graphically presented in figure 3. This graph shows that the current-voltage relationship is not linear. When the membrane potential was more positive than the holding potential, the resistance dropped to 3 MΩ. This increase in the membrane conductance is expected to be a voltage-dependent K conductance.

The inward current of the outer hair cell was observed (fig. 4). The outward current was completely blocked by both 30 mM TEA of Ca solution and 130 mM Cs of Cs solution. These inward currents disappeared 15 min after the rupture of the membrane patch. 35 ms after the start of a voltage pulse, the inward currents were corrected by subtracting leakage current and the current-voltage relationship was obtained (fig. 5). Voltage-dependent inactivation of this inward current was observed at about 10 mV. Time-dependent inactivation was not observed.

Whole Cell Recording under the Current Clamp

Changes of the membrane potential in Na solution were recorded by the current clamp method. Square steps of the depolarizing current were injected in the hair cell during the current clamp.

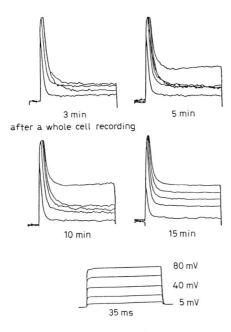

3 min   5 min

after a whole cell recording

10 min   15 min

80 mV

40 mV

5 mV

35 ms

Fig. 4. Inward currents of a cochlear outer hair cell (Vh-50 mV).

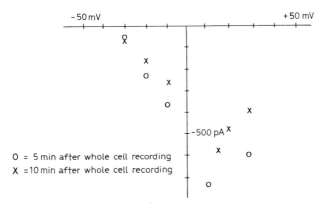

− 50 mV   + 50 mV

−500 pA

O = 5 min after whole cell recording

X = 10 min after whole cell recording

Fig. 5. Current-voltage relationship for the cochlear outer hair cell. The current was measured 35 ms after the start of a voltage step.

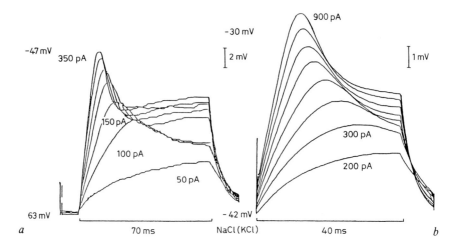

Fig. 6. Changes of membrane potential produced by current pulses. *a* Saccular hair cell. *b* Cochlear outer hair cell.

The membrane potential increased up to 10 mV when the current over the threshold was given. Then the membrane potential decreased although the depolarizing current was injected (fig. 6). The duration of the increase in the membrane potential was almost constant and was about 10 ms. The peak voltage was not linear to the depolarizing currents.

Discussion

The resting potential of the hair cell has been investigated by various methods. The intracellular recording technique has been most frequently utilized. Especially in the cochlear outer and inner hair cells the resting potential is a primary component for its frequency tuning [6, 8].

Physiologically a hair cell is exposed to two different fluids. Once the hair cell is dissociated, this ionic environment is lost. Yet, the resting potential in Na solution whose concentration is similar to the perilymphatic fluid was comparable to the measurements by the intracellular recordings.

Ionic currents which had been found in a hair cell are Ca current, Ca-activated K current, transient K current and anomalous rectifier K current [7]. In our experiment the outward rectification which occurred more positive than –50 mV was blocked by 30 mM TEA of the external solution and 130 mM Cs of the internal solution. This confirmed that the outward rectification was a voltage-dependent K conductance. Anomalous rectification [1, 7] could not be recorded. The inward current recorded by blocking the outward current is probably Ca current, since no Na current is found in a hair cell [1, 5, 7]. Ca current is reportedly not inactivated [5]. But in our experiment Ca current showed a voltage-dependent inactivation just as found in a rod inner segment of the retinal cell [4].

The receptor potential at least up to 15 mV reportedly can be produced in the hair cell by directly stimulating its hair bundle. The action potential with the amplitude of about 40 mV was also observed [2]. The amplitude of the membrane potential under the current clamp is about 10 mV, suggesting that this is a receptor potential. In our whole cell clamp experiment action potential was not so far observed. However, the action potential had been evoked in the retinal rod inner segments [4]. Further study is needed to determine if the action potential can occur in the inner ear hair cell under different experimental conditions.

References

1   Goldstein, A.J.; Hudspeth, A.J.: Voltage- and ion-dependent conductance in solitary vertebrate hair cells. Nature *304:* 538–541 (1983).
2   Hudspeth, A.J.; Cory, D.P.: Sensitivity, polarity and conductance change in the response of vertebrate hair cells to controlled mechanical stimuli. Proc. natn. Acad. Sci. USA *74:* 2407–2411 (1977).
3   Hodgkin, A.L.; Huxley, A.F.: A quantitative description of membrane current and its application to conductance and excitation in nerve. J. Physiol. *117:* 500–544 (1952).
4   Bader, C.R.; et al.: Voltage-activated and calcium-activated currents studied in solitary rod inner segments from the salamander retina. J. Physiol. *331:* 253–284 (1982).
5   Cory, D.P.; Hudspeth, A.J.: Ionic basis of the receptor potential in a vertebrate hair cell. Nature *281:* 675–677 (1979).
6   Russell, I.J.; Sellick, P.M.: Intracellular studies of hair cells in the mammalian cochlea. J. Physiol. *284:* 261–290 (1978).
7   Ohmori, H.: Studies of ionic currents in the isolated vestibular hair cell of the chick. J. Physiol. *350:* 561–581 (1984).
8   Dallos, P.; Santos-Sacchi, J.; Flock, Å.: Intracellular recordings from cochlear outer hair cells. Science *218:* 582–584 (1982).

Y. Harada, MD, Department of Otolaryngology, Hiroshima University,
School of Medicine, 1-2-3 Kasumi, Minamiku, Hiroshima 734 (Japan)

Adv. Oto-Rhino-Laryng., vol. 41, pp. 14–19 (Karger, Basel 1988)

HRP Morphology of Functionally Identified Vestibular Type I Neurons in the Cat

Tohru Ohgaki[a], *Ian S. Curthoys*[b], *Charles H. Markham*[a]

[a] Department of Neurology, UCLA School of Medicine, Los Angeles, Calif., USA;
[b] Department of Psychology, University of Sydney, Sydney, NSW, Australia

Introduction

Vestibular type I neurons receive input from horizontal canal primary afferents projected to the abducens nucleus and elsewhere, and participate in the vestibulo-ocular reflex. In this study, physiologically identified type I neurons were stained using a horse-radish peroxidase (HRP) intracellular staining technique to analyze their morphological character.

Method

Horizontal canal secondary type I neurons in ketamine anesthetized cats were identified by their characteristic firing pattern related to horizontal rotation and by short latency activation on electrical stimulation of the vestibular nerve. (Only those with a relatively fixed latency of less than 1.4 ms are considered here.) Axons and occasionally cell bodies were penetrated by microelectrodes filled with 6% HRP in 0.05 M Tris:HCl, 0.2 M KCl buffer (pH = 8.6). HRP was injected iontophoretically. 200-ms pulses of 10–20 nA depolarizing constant current were passed through the electrode at 2.5 pulses/s for 10–20 min. After 10–24 h, the animals were perfused transcardially with 0.1 M phosphate buffer solution followed by a mixture of 1% glutaraldehyde and 2% paraformaldehyde in 0.1 M phosphate buffer (pH = 7.4). The brain was cut in 100-μm horizontal or coronal sections. The sections were treated for HRP using the diaminobenzidine method [1], placed on slides and counterstained. Each satisfactorily stained neuron was reconstructed at a magnification of ×400 or ×1,000, using a Zeiss microscope equipped with a camera lucida drawing attachment.

Result

Forty-four cell bodies or axons in 28 cats were stained. Nineteen neurons projected to the contralateral side of the brain stem, and 21 neurons projected to the ipsilateral side. In 4 neurons, only the cell bodies and dendrites were stained.

Type I neurons were located in the rostral portion of the medial vestibular nucleus. The cell bodies were big and had rather elongated shapes and rich dendritic arborization.

In contralaterally projecting neurons, stem axons crossed the midline and bifurcated into rostral and caudal branches in the contralateral medial longitudinal fasciculus (MLF). Figure 1 shows a representative example. Three tertiary collaterals arose close to the bifurcation and distributed many terminals in a relatively wide area in the contralateral abducens nucleus. Some of these collaterals in the abducens nucleus projected further to the contralateral medial vestibular nucleus. A tertiary collateral arose from the main rostral branch and terminated in the contralateral MLF. Sometimes a tertiary collateral arose from the caudal branch and projected to the contra-lateral nucleus praepositus hypoglossi (PH) (not shown here). The main rostral and caudal branches filled with HRP to a length of about 5 mm and were then lost from view. All contralaterally projecting neurons showed almost the same projecting pattern.

On the other hand, ipsilateral projecting vestibular neurons had a much more varied projecting pattern. Five representative neurons are shown in figure 2. Neuron A projected only to the abducens nucleus and had no further ascending or descending branches. Primary axons of neurons B and C entered the abducens nucleus and had terminal distribution there. Each had branches projecting to the nucleus reticularis pontis caudalis immediately rostral to the abducens nucleus, and had caudal branches projecting to PH. C also had collaterals which projected to the nucleus raphe pontis caudalis where omnipause neurons exist, and a large rostrally projecting branch.

Neurons D and E had thick descending stem axons which entered in ipsilateral MLF and were lost from view at the level of the hypoglossal nucleus. Neuron D had collaterals which projected to the abducens nucleus but neuron E did not project to the abducens. Both D and E had collaterals which projected to PH and the paramedian reticular nucleus, and both seemed to be medial vestibulospinal tract neurons. All ipsilateral vestibular neurons except E distributed to a relatively limited region in the ipsilateral abducens nucleus in contrast to the contralateral projecting vestibular neurons.

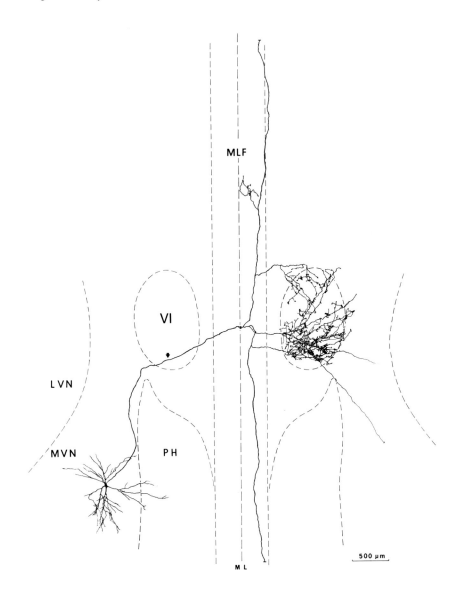

Fig. 1. Contralateral projection vestibular type I neuron. Arrow shows the injection point which was in the ipsilateral abducens nucleus. VI = Abducens nucleus; LVN = lateral vestibular nucleus; MVN = medial vestibular nucleus; MLF = medial longitudinal fasciculus; PH = nucleus praepositus hypoglossi.

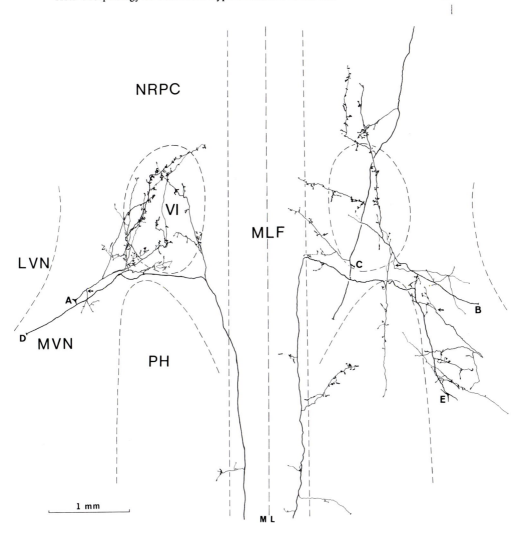

Fig. 2. Five examples of ipsilateral projection vestibular type I neurons. Arrow shows the collaterals which project to the ipsilateral medial vestibular nucleus. NRPC = Nucleus reticularis pontis caudalis.

Another important characteristic of many of the ipsilateral projecting neurons was their extensive terminal arborization in the medial vestibular nucleus close to their cells of origin.

Discussion

Electrophysiological studies [2, 4] have shown that there are excitatory and inhibitory type I neurons and that the former project to contralateral abducens nucleus and the latter to ipsilateral abducens nucleus. According to these findings, it may be concluded that the contralateral projecting neurons we observed are the excitatory type I neurons and that ipsilateral vestibular neurons, except neurons similar to E, are the inhibitory type I neurons. The contralateral projecting neurons are very similar to those shown by Ishizuka et al. [3] and McCrea et al. [5] using the HRP technique. The ipsilateral projecting type I neurons shown here as B or C have been previously described by Ishizuka et al. [3], and E by McCrea et al. [5]. A and D appear to be newly described in the present study.

The contralateral projecting neurons not only projected to the abducens nucleus but also to contralateral PH, raphe and medial vestibular nucleus. The last probably constitutes the main vestibular commissural pathway linking second order horizontal canal neurons via intercalated inhibitory type II neurons [6]. Inhibitory vestibular neurons had more varied projection patterns. Some projected to areas containing pause neurons and premotor burst neurons and may therefore be involved in the genesis of quick eye movements. Some inhibitory vestibular neurons had extensive terminations in the ipsilateral medial vestibular nucleus; we suggest these may terminate on type II neurons and act to suppress their activity during ipsilateral rotation.

References

1   Adams, J.C.: Heavy metal intensification of DAB-based HRP reaction product. J. Histochem. Cytochem. *29:* 775 (1981).
2   Baker, R.G.; Mano, N.; Shimazu, H.: Postsynaptic potentials in abducens motoneurons induced by vestibular stimulation. Brain Res. *15:* 577–580 (1969).
3   Ishizuka, N.; Mannen, H.; Sasaki, S.; Shimazu, H.: Axonal branches and terminations in the cat abducens nucleus of secondary vestibular neurons in the horizontal canal system. Neurosci. Lett. *16:* 143–148 (1980).

4   Maeda, M.; Shimazu, H.; Shinoda, Y.: Nature of synaptic events in cat abducens motoneurons at slow and quick phase of vestibular nystagmus. J. Neurophysiol. *35:* 279–296 (1972).

5   McCrea, R.A.; Yoshida, K.; Berthoz, A.; Baker, R.: Eye movement related activity and morphology of second order vestibular neurons terminating in the cat abducens nucleus. Exp. Brain Res. *40:* 468–473 (1980).

6   Shimazu, H.; Precht, W.: Inhibition of central vestibular neurons from the contralateral labyrinth and its mediating pathway. J. Neurophysiol. *29:* 467–492 (1966).

Tohru Ohgaki, MD, Department of Neurology, UCLA School of Medicine, Los Angeles, CA 90024-1769 (USA)

Adv. Oto-Rhino-Laryng., vol. 41, pp. 20–24 (Karger, Basel 1988)

Physiological Characteristics of the Primary Horizontal Canal Neurons in Guinea Pigs: Response Difference between Alert and Anesthetized Animals

Toshiaki Yagi, Hiroshi Ueno

Department of Otolaryngology, Nippon Medical School, Bunkyo-ku, Tokyo, Japan

Introduction

The physiological characteristics of the semicircular canal primary neurons have been intensively studied in many species. An average resting rate of 32.4 spikes/s was reported by Yagi et al. [1] in anesthetized cats. A clearly higher average resting rate of 59.2 spikes/s was, however, demonstrated by Ezure et al. [2] in alert cats. It thus seems quite important to ascertain the effect of the general anesthesia used when discussing the function of the vestibular efferent system. In the present study, we accordingly investigated the spontaneous activity and the response to sinusoidal rotation of the primary horizontal semicircular canal neurons in alert guinea pigs as compared with those we previously reported in anesthetized guinea pigs [3].

Subjects and Methods

Nineteen albino guinea pigs were used in this study. The animals received the ultra short-acting anesthetic, thiopental sodium, intraperitoneally. After a tracheostomy, they were placed on a pendular rotation turntable. Before recovering from anesthesia, a right parieto-occipital craniotomy was performed and the spinal cord was transected at C_1. The guinea pigs were artificially respirated and no anesthetics, except for one locally applied to the wound edge, was given for the remainder of the experiment. Portions of flocculus and paraflocculus were aspirated to expose the primary neurons for recording. The area of Scarpa's ganglion was identified and a glass microelectrode filled with 2 M NaCl was inserted into the ganglion for recording the extracellular activities from single neurons.

Results

One hundred and thirty-five horizontal semicircular canal neurons were analyzed in this experiment. The neurons had an average resting rate of 47.3 spikes/s with a standard deviation (SD) of 21.1 and a range of 2.2–113.6 spikes/s. These values were significantly higher than those from anesthetized guinea pigs (p <0.01) which had an average rate of 39.1 ± 20.5 spikes/s and a range of 1.9–90.9 spikes/s (n = 121). The significant level here and elsewhere in this paper was determined using the two-tailed t-test.

The regularity of the units was determined using the coefficient of variation (CV). The average CV for the horizontal canal neurons was 0.299 with an SD of 0.270 and a range of 0.032–0.956. These values were no different from those of the anesthetized guinea pigs. From the CV values, the neurons were classified into three groups according to the cat experiment classification: regular, intermediate, and irregular firing units [4]. The incidence of the regular units was slightly higher than that in the anesthetized animals. The average resting rates, ± SD, of the regular, intermediate, and irregular units in alert guinea pigs were 55.9 ± 10.2, 50.0 ± 23.0, and 17.9 ± 10.3 spikes/s, respectively. The resting rate of the intermediate units was significantly higher than the 39.1 ± 16.9 spikes/s noted in the anesthetized animals. In the anesthetized guinea pigs, these three neuron groups were from different populations (p <0.01). In the alert guinea pigs, however, the resting rate of the intermediate neurons featured higher resting rate, so that no statistically significant difference was found in the resting rates between the regular and intermediate groups.

The gain and phase of the horizontal canal neurons to sinusoidal stimulation were examined. The average gain from a total of 66 units tested at 0.3 Hz was 0.42 spikes/s/deg/s with an SD of 0.33. This value was the same as that of anesthetized guinea pigs. The mean gains, ± SD, of the regular, intermediate, and irregular units at the same stimulus frequency were 0.22 ± 0.20 (n − 27), 0.57 ± 0.35 (n = 23), and 0.52 ± 0.28 (n − 12), respectively. No statistical difference occurred between these values and those of anesthetized guinea pigs.

The average phase lag to the acceleration at 0.3 Hz was 57.3 degrees with an SD of 20.7 (n = 67). This value was clearly smaller than that from the anesthetized guinea pigs where the means and SD of the phase lag was 75.3 ± 24.3 (n = 56). The means of the phase lag in the regular, intermediate, and irregular unit groups were 65.4 (n = 22), 58.8 (n = 24), and 55.0 (n = 15), respectively. These values were significantly smaller than those from the

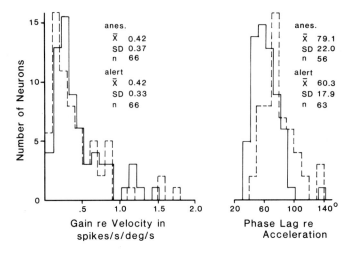

Fig. 1. Histograms of the gains and phase lag at 0.3 Hz stimulation of recorded neurons in alert (solid line) and anesthetized (broken line) guinea pigs.

anesthetized guinea pigs. Figure 1 shows the histograms of the gain (a) and phase lag (b) of the recorded neurons in the alert (solid line) and anesthetized (broken line) guinea pigs at a frequency of 0.3 Hz.

The number of cutoff neurons at 0.3 Hz stimulation in alert guinea pigs was only one (1.5%) among 67 neurons recorded. This is clearly a lower incidence than that recorded in anesthetized guinea pigs where the number of cutoff neurons was seven (10.9%) out of 64 neurons.

Discussion

Two possible effective sites of general anesthesia which modulate primary vestibular afferent activities could be considered. One is the afferent nerve itself and the other is the vestibular efferent neurons in the brain stem and other related structures such as the brain stem reticular formation. The barbiturate, however, manages the excitability of the central nervous system, especially the cerebral cortex and the reticular activating system, rather than the peripheral nervous system. Thus, the effect of barbiturate on the afferent nerve itself seems to be a less important candidate of the possible affected sites.

The origin of the efferent vestibular neurons has been identified in the brain stem [5]. The functional role of the vestibular efferent system, however, remains controversial. Experimental evidence of the efferent system demonstrating a weak inhibitory effect on the afferent activities has been reported in frogs and cats [6, 7]. On the other hand, Keller [8] stated that the vestibular efferent system has no effect on the activities of the primary semicircular canal neurons from his experimental results using alert and anesthetized monkeys. Recently, the increase in spontaneous discharge rate and the rise of gains of the primary vestibular neurons were reported by Goldberg and Fernandez [9], using electric stimulation applied to the efferent vestibular neuronal pool in the brain stem of monkeys. Furthermore, Highstein and Baker [10] stated that the efferent vestibular neurons were spontaneously active and increased their frequency of discharge when the fish they were using were behaviorally aroused. This caused a subsequent increase in the spontaneous discharge rate of the primary vestibular afferent neurons.

The present experiment revealed an increase in the spontaneous discharge and the shortening of the phase lag to the angular acceleration in the alert guinea pigs. In addition to these results, an extremely small number of cutoff neurons, one out of 67 neurons at 0.3 Hz stimulation, were found in the alert guinea pigs. The decrease in the number of cutoff neurons was probably due to the increase in the spontaneous discharge level. This may expand the dynamic range and raise the linearity of the function of the semicircular canal system. Thus, the vestibular efferent system is speculated to help control the generation of the functional distortion of the semicircular canal endorgans when the mechanical stimulation is transformed to the neural activities.

References

1   Yagi, T.; Simpson, N.E.; Markham, C.H.: The relationship of conduction velocity to other physiological properties of the cat's horizontal canal neurons. Exp. Brain Res. *30:* 587–600 (1977).
2   Ezure, K.; Schor, R.H.; Yoshida, K.: The response of horizontal semicircular canal afferents to sinusoidal rotation in the cat. Exp. Brain Res. *33:* 27–39 (1978).
3   Yagi, T.; Ueno. H.; Yamaguchi, J.: Physiological characteristics of the primary horizontal canal neurons in guinea pigs; in Graham, Kemink, The vestibular system, pp. 141–147 (Raven Press, New York 1987).

4   Estes, M.S.; Blanks, R.H.I.; Markham, C.H.: Physiologic characteristics of vestibular first-order canal neurons in the cat. I. Response plane determination and resting characteristics. J. Neurophysiol. *38:* 1232–1249 (1975).

5   Gacek, R.R.; Lyon, M.: The localization of vestibular efferent neurons in the kitten with horseradish peroxidase. Acta oto-lar. *77:* 92–101 (1974).

6   Linás, R.; Precht, W.: The inhibitory vestibular efferent system and its relation to the cerebellum in the frog. Exp. Brain Res. *9:* 16–29 (1969).

7   Dieringer, A.; Blanks, R.H.I.; Precht, W.: Cat efferent vestibular system: weak suppression of primary afferent activity. Neurosci. Lett. *5:* 285–290 (1977).

8   Keller, E.L.: Behavior of horizontal semicircular canal afferents in alert monkeys during vestibular and optokinetic stimulation. Exp. Brain Res. *24:* 459–471 (1976).

9   Goldberg, J.M.; Fernandez, C.: Efferent vestibular system in the squirrel monkey: anatomical location and influence on afferent activity. J. Neurophysiol. *43:* 986–1025 (1980).

10 Highstein, S.M.; Baker, R.: Action of the efferent vestibular system on primary afferent in the toad fish, opsanus tau. J. Neurophysiol. *54:* 370–384 (1985).

Toshiaki Yagi, MD, Department of Otolaryngology, Nippon Medical School,
1-1-5 Sendagi, Bunkyo-ku, Tokyo 113 (Japan)

Adv. Oto-Rhino-Laryng., vol. 41, pp. 25–30 (Karger, Basel 1988)

The Effects of Ethyl Alcohol on the Non-Linear Characteristics of Visual-Vestibular Interaction

G.R. Barnes, R.D. Eason, A.J. Eldridge

RAF Institute of Aviation Medicine, Farnborough, Hants, England

Introduction

When the human subject attempts to suppress the vestibulo-ocular reflex (VOR) by fixation of a head-fixed target during whole-body rotation, two types of non-linearity may be identified in the response: (a) prediction [Barnes, 1987] and (b) velocity saturation [Barnes and Edge, 1983]. In the experiments described here we have investigated the effect of ethanol, which is known to impair VOR suppression, on these non-linear characteristics.

Method

Subjects were seated on a turntable with head and body firmly fixed to the supporting structure. The turntable was oscillated about the yaw axis so as to stimulate the lateral semi-circular canals and thereby induce lateral eye movements. In the first experiment the pseudo-random motion stimulus was composed of four harmonically unrelated sinusoids of equal peak angular velocity ($\pm$ 17.5 deg/s). The three lowest frequencies of the stimulus remained constant (0.11, 0.24 and 0.37 Hz) whilst the highest frequency (F_4) was varied from 0.39 to 2.08 Hz. Eye movements were recorded in three visual stimulus conditions: (a) in darkness, whilst the subjects carried out a simple auditory pitch discrimination task; (b) whilst the subjects attempted to suppress the VOR by fixation of a target which was rigidly fixed to the turntable, and (c) in darkness, whilst the subjects attempted to suppress the VOR by fixation of an imaginary head-fixed target. In the second experiment turntable motion was a low frequency (0.05 Hz) sinusoid of peak velocity $\pm$ 120 deg/s. Eye movements recorded in darkness were compared with those evoked during suppression of the VOR by fixation of a head-fixed target in three visual stimulus conditions in which there was (a) no background (DRK), (b) a full field striped background which moved with the turntable (HF), and (c) the same background fixed in space (EF). In both experiments eye movements were recorded by an infra-red limbus tracking method. Subjects performed the experimental tasks in a control condition and 30 min after ingestion of a dose of alcohol. Dose level was 2.1 ml/kg body weight administered in the form of equal measures of vodka and orange juice. Mean pre-trial blood alcohol concentration was 80 mg/100 ml in the first experiment and 75 mg/100 ml in the second.

The Effects of Ethanol on the Predictive Mechanisms of VOR Suppression

The Effects of Ethanol on the Predictive Mechanisms of VOR Suppression

VOR Response in the Dark. The gain and phase of the slow-phase component of the vestibulo-ocular reflex were not significantly modified by the frequency content of the motion stimulus, nor were they significantly changed by the effects of ethanol. Mean gain for the 8 subjects was 0.57 in the control condition and 0.54 in the alcohol condition.

Visual Suppression of the VOR. When the subjects attempted to suppress the VOR by fixation of the head-fixed target in both the control and alcohol conditions the degree of suppression achieved was significantly diminished ($p < 0.001$ by analysis of variance) as the frequency of the highest frequency component was increased. The effectiveness of suppression may be assessed by calculation of VOR suppression gain (G_s), that is the ratio between the eye velocity during suppression and that recorded in darkness (fig. 1). In the control condition, when F_4 was 0.39 Hz mean VOR suppression gain averaged over the three lowest frequencies was 0.10, but as F_4 increased to 2.08 Hz mean gain for the same three frequencies increased to 0.30 (fig. 1). Under the influence of alcohol VOR suppression gain also increased significantly ($p < 0.001$) as F_4 was increased, but was significantly ($p < 0.001$) greater than in the control condition for all values of F_4, the mean gain for the three lowest frequencies increasing from 0.27 to 0.56 as F_4 increased from 0.39 to 2.08 Hz (fig. 1). The phase associated with the gain of VOR suppression exhibited a phase lag at the lowest frequency (0.11 Hz) which changed to phase advance at the highest frequency (2.08 Hz). Under the influence of alcohol there was significantly less phase lag at the lowest frequency and less phase lead at the highest frequency.

Non-Visual Suppression of the VOR. When subjects attempted to suppress the VOR by fixation of an imagined head-fixed target in darkness, the

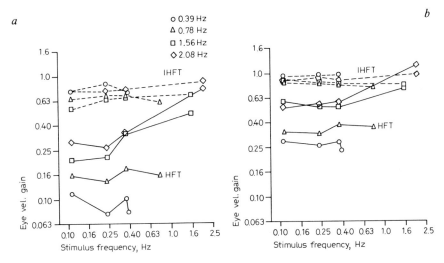

Fig. 1. VOR suppression gain (i.e. the ratio of eye velocity during suppression to eye velocity in the dark) in response to pseudo-random angular head motion stimuli composed of four sinusoids. The three lowest frequencies were maintained at 0.11, 0.24 and 0.37 Hz, whilst the highest frequency was varied from 0.39 to 2.08 Hz. HFT = Real head-fixed target; IHFT = imagined head-fixed target. *a* Control condition; *b* alcohol condition.

frequency content of the stimulus had no significant effect on the degree of suppression achieved. However, significantly less suppression was achieved under the influence of alcohol than in the control condition. Mean VOR suppression gain increased from 0.72 in the control condition to 0.90 under the influence of alcohol.

The Effects of Ethanol on the Velocity Saturation Effects of VOR Suppression

VOR Response in the Dark. As in the first experiment, ethanol had no significant effect on the gain and phase of the VOR recorded in the dark. Mean gain for the 6 subjects was 0.44 in the control condition and 0.38 under the influence of alcohol.

Visual Suppression of the VOR. When the subjects attempted to suppress the VOR by fixation of a head-fixed target, the degree of suppression achieved was significantly ($p < 0.001$) less under the influence of alcohol than

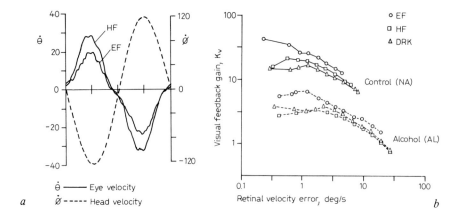

Fig. 2. *a* Mean single cycle slow-phase eye velocity and head velocity trajectories (in units of deg/s) representing the average of four cycles of sinusoidal oscillation at 0.05 Hz while viewing a head-fixed target under the influence of alcohol. *b* Visual feedback gain (K_v) as a function of retinal velocity error (i.e. slow-phase eye velocity) during VOR suppression by fixation of a head-fixed target under control and alcohol conditions. Symbols refer to visual background conditions: DRK = darkness; EF = earth-fixed stripes; HF = head-fixed stripes.

in the control condition. Eye velocity gain was also significantly ($p < 0.05$) less when the stationary structured background was present than when a blank background or head-fixed structured background was used, in accord with the findings of Guedry et al. [1979]. In the non-alcohol condition mean VOR suppression gain rose from 0.07 in the presence of the earth-fixed background to 0.12 when there was no background present. Corresponding gains for the alcohol condition were 0.39 and 0.55.

Non-Linear Characteristics of Visual Suppression of the VOR. During each cycle of stimulation the degree of suppression achieved decreased as the velocity of the stimulus increased from 0 to 120 deg/s, as revealed by the cycle-by-cycle average shown in figure 2a. The effectiveness of suppression may be assessed by calculation of the VOR suppression gain (G_s) in the manner described above. If it is assumed, as in a previous publication [Barnes and Edge, 1983], that this suppression is achieved through a visual feedback mechanism with retinal velocity sensitivity K_v, the relationship between G_s and K_v may be expressed in the form $G_s = 1/(1 + K_v)$. The results shown in figure 2a indicate that as head velocity increases G_s also increases and that, therefore, K_v decreases. The calculated values of K_v for different velocity levels in the stimulus waveform have been plotted in figure 2b as a function of retinal velocity error (i.e. slow-phase eye velocity in this instance). From this it can be seen that K_v is fairly constant at low velocity (up to 2 deg/s) but then decreases progressively as retinal velocity error increases in the manner described previously [Barnes and Edge, 1983]. This non-linear effect was observed for all stimulus conditions, although under the influence of alcohol the value of K_v decreased by a factor of approximately 5–6 when compared with the control condition. It is also evident that in both the control and alcohol conditions K_v remained higher in the presence of the earth-fixed, structured background than for the other two visual background conditions.

Discussion

The effects of ethanol described here are very similar to those found in previous experiments, not only for visual suppression of the VOR, but also for pursuit [Baloh et al., 1979; Barnes et al., 1985]. It is now well established that visual suppression of the VOR and pursuit share a number of common features, including the two non-linear characteristics described here (Barnes and Crombie, 1985; Barnes, 1987]. Moreover, experiments in which passive [Barnes and Crombie, 1985; Barnes, 1987] or transient [Miles and Kawano, 1986] stimulation of the oculomotor system have been used have indicated that prediction, velocity saturation and the stationary background effects are all features of the basic feedback mechanism responsible for the visual control of eye movement.

The results of the two experiments described here indicate that the salient features of these non-linear characteristics are not modified by the effects of alcohol. Rather, it is the efficacy of the final inhibitory process which appears to be impaired even during non-visual VOR suppression.

References

Baloh, R.W.; Sharma, S.; Moskowitz, H.; Griffith, R.: Effect of alcohol and marijuana on eye movements. Aviat. Space envir. Med. *50:* 18–23 (1979).
Barnes, G.R.: Head-eye co-ordination: the role of prediction in visual-vestibular interaction; in Pompeiano, Allum, Vestibular control of posture and locomotion. Prog. Brain Res. (in press 1987).

Barnes, G.R.; Crombie, J.W.: The interaction of conflicting retinal motion stimuli in oculomotor control. Exp. Brain Res. *59:* 548–558 (1985).

Barnes, G.R.; Crombie, J.W.; Edge, A.: The effects of ethanol on visual-vestibular interaction during active and passive head movements. Aviat. Space envir. Med. *56:* 695–701 (1985).

Barnes, G.R.; Edge, A.: Non-linear effects in suppression of vestibular nystagmus. Exp. Brain Res. *52:* 9–19 (1983).

Guedry, F.E.; Lentz, J.M.; Jell, R.M.: Visual-vestibular interactions. I. Influence of peripheral vision on suppression of the vestibulo-ocular reflex and visual acuity. Aviat. Space envir. Med. *50:* 205–211 (1979).

Miles, F.A.; Kawano, K.: Short-latency ocular following responses of monkey. 1. Dependence on temporospatial properties of visual input. J. Neurophysiol. *56:* 1321 (1986).

G.R. Barnes, PhD, RAF Institute of Aviation Medicine, Farnborough, Hants, GU14 6SZ (England)

Adv. Oto-Rhino-Laryng., vol. 41, pp. 31–35 (Karger, Basel 1988)

Evaluation of VOR Function with Gaze Stabilization

Masahiro Takahashi, Naomi Tsujita, Ikuyo Akiyama

Department of Otolaryngology, Tokyo Women's Medical College, Tokyo, Japan

Introduction

Since low-frequency rotation tests, being reported to have high diagnostic values [1], differ considerably from the situations in daily life, we must examine gaze-stabilizing functions during head rotations to evaluate the vestibular-ocular reflex (VOR). The purpose of this paper is to clarify the relationship between VOR functions and gaze functions by analyzing the results obtained in subjects with different status of VOR function.

Subjects and Methods

We reported on five different groups: 20 normal adults, 20 normal children aged 3–10 (5.8 on average), 15 patients with cerebellar dysfunction, 3 patients with bilateral loss of labyrinthine function, and 5 patients with unilateral loss of labyrinthine function, who were examined at an average of 20.4 days after onset.

The subjects were sinusoidally rotated by an electrically driven chair at an amplitude of 40° at frequencies of 0.2, 0.33, 0.67 and 0.85 Hz [2]. Rotation tests were done under three different visual conditions: with the subject performing mental arithmetic in the dark, with the subject visually fixating on a target on the wall, and with the subject visually fixating on a head-fixed target [3].

Head movements were recorded by a gyrosensor affixed to the head. Horizontal eye movements were recorded with a DC electro-oculograph. They were electrically added to the head movements to ascertain gaze movements in space. For analysis of the recordings, the ratio of the maximum slow-phase eye velocity to the corresponding head rotation velocity (gain) was manually obtained by averaging measurements on the most stable recordings.

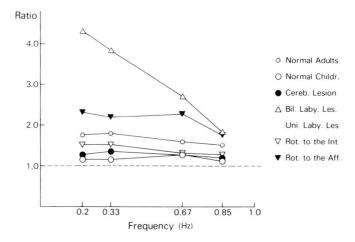

Fig. 1. The ratio of the gain under the spatially fixed target condition to VOR gain.

Results

VOR gain showed a large variation in normal adults as well as in patients
with cerebellar lesions. Normal children presented large VOR gain values
(0.92 ± 0.12 at 0.85 Hz) resembling the values obtained in patients with
cerebellar lesions (0.88 ± 0.19), both of which differed significantly from
those in normal adults (0.69 ± 0.15). Patients with unilateral labyrinthine
lesion presented a remarkable directional difference in the gain (0.84 and
0.38 on average).

Under fixation on a target on the wall, mean gain values were accurately
maintained at unity not only in normal adults and children, but in patients
with unilateral labyrinthine lesion upon rotations to the intact side. Patients
with cerebellar lesions manifested a significantly larger variance of the gain
(1.02 ± 0.12 at 0.85 Hz) than normal adults (1.01 ± 0.04). In patients with
bilateral labyrinthine lesions and patients with unilateral lesion upon
rotations to the affected side, gaze fixation became worse with an increase in
rotation frequency (0.26 and 0.38, respectively, at 0.85 Hz).

The mean ratio of the gain under the spatially fixed target condition to
the VOR gain differed markedly among different subject groups at low
frequencies: 1.17 at 0.2 Hz in children to 4.32 in bilateral labyrinthine lesion
(fig. 1). However, even in patients with labyrinthine lesion, the ratio con-
verged on values less than 2.0 as the frequency increased: 1.85 at 0.85 Hz in

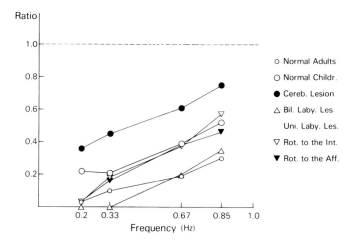

Fig. 2. The ratio of the gain under the head-fixed target condition to VOR gain.

bilateral lesion and 1.75 upon rotations to the affected side in unilateral lesion. Theoretical approximation of the ratio at higher frequencies suggested that gain values under the spatially fixed target condition corresponded with those in the dark at 1.0–2.5 Hz.

Under fixation on a head-fixed target, gaze stabilization became worse with increased oscillation frequency and it varied markedly at high frequencies among different subject groups. Gaze fixation was disturbed even at lower frequencies in cerebellar lesions. Children showed gain values (0.47 ± 0.17 at 0.85 Hz) significantly different from both those in normal adults (0.20 ± 0.08) and those in cerebellar lesions (0.66 ± 0.21).

Although the ratio of the gain under the head-fixed target condition to the VOR gain varied from 0.30 in normal adults to 0.75 in cerebellar lesions, it increased lineally with an increase in the rotation frequency (fig. 2). The approximate values of the ratio of the gain at higher frequencies indicated that VOR will be no more suppressed by gaze at frequencies higher than 1.3–3.0 Hz.

Discussion and Conclusions

We could discriminate three different strategies realizing spatial gaze fixation: a little adjustment of the gain in the light combined with large VOR gain values (cerebellar dysfunction and children), internal amplification of the gain by releasing the VOR from the inhibitory regulation (normal adults), and recalibration with high magnifications of small VOR gain values (labyrinthine lesion) [4, 5]. The dual control of the VOR gain in normal adults makes the system adaptable to variable internal and external environments. The large VOR gain values observed in cerebellar lesions and children may result from a decline and an immaturity, respectively, in the inhibitory regulation of the VOR, which is not directly related to gaze-stabilizing function, but evolutionally related to acquisition of the function to gaze at a spatially moving target during head rotations.

A decline in the ability of fixation-induced suppression on the VOR could increase VOR gain in normal adults. Preliminary study indicated that drinking alcohol (0.43 ml/kg) after hunger not only decreased fixation-induced suppression, but also increased VOR gain; the higher the alcohol concentration in the expired air, the worse the fixation-induced suppression. In addition, the smaller the VOR gain before drinking, the larger the alteration in the VOR gain.

Since labyrinthine dysfunction itself did not affect fixation-induced suppression, a decline in the ability in the early unilateral lesion may be produced by an acute loss of balance between bilateral VOR arcs, which possibly produces bias on the suppressive mechanism.

From the frequency-dependent characteristics of the ratio of the gain in the light to the VOR gain, theoretical approximation indicates that VOR can be neither amplified nor suppressed by gaze at oscillation frequencies higher than at least 3.0 Hz. From the present study, we can say that quantification of gaze effects on the VOR under rotations at low to high frequencies offer more valuable information about the regulation of the VOR than measurement of VOR gain under extreme high-frequency rotations to eliminate gaze effects [6].

References

1   Hess, K.; et al.: Rotational testing in patients with bilateral peripheral vestibular disease. Laryngoscope 95: 85–88 (1985).
2   Takahashi, M.; et al.: Compensatory eye movement and gaze fixation upon passive head-and-body rotation and active head rotation. Archs Oto-Rhino-Lar. 238: 157–166 (1983).
3   Takahashi, M.; et al.: Studies of the vestibulo-ocular reflex and visual-vestibular interactions during active head movements. Acta oto-lar. 90: 115–124 (1980).

4 Takahashi, M.; et al.: Compensatory eye movement and gaze fixation during active head rotation in patients with labyrinthine disorders. Ann. Otol. Rhinol. Lar. *90:* 241–245 (1981).
5 Takahashi, M.; et al.: Recovery of vestibulo-ocular reflex and gaze disturbance in patients with unilateral loss of labyrinthine function. Ann. Otol. Rhinol. Lar. *93:* 170–175 (1984).
6 Hydén, D.; et al.: Quantification of slow compensatory eye movements in patients with bilateral vestibular loss. Acta oto-lar. *96:* 199–206 (1983).

Masahiro Takahashi, MD, Department of Otolaryngology, Yokohama Municipal Citizen's Hospital, 56 Okazawacho, Hodogayaku, Yokohamashi 240 (Japan)

Adv. Oto-Rhino-Laryng., vol. 41, pp. 36–39 (Karger, Basel 1988)

Developmental Modulation of Vestibular-Ocular Function

Edward M. Ornitz, Vicente Honrubia

Division of Mental Retardation and Child Psychiatry and Division of Head and Neck Surgery, UCLA School of Medicine, Brain Research Institute, Los Angeles, Calif., USA

In comparison to adults, infants in the early months of life have larger gains and shorter time constants of the vestibulo-ocular reflex (VOR) [Ornitz, in press]. The VOR gain decreases and the time constant lengthens during childhood, approaching adult values after 10 years of age. It has been suggested [Ornitz, in press] that the developmental changes in the VOR cannot be attributed to increasing experience with *vestibular* input since repeated vestibular stimulation reduces rather than increases the time constant of the VOR [Jager and Henn, 1981].

Visual experience associated with maturation of the visual system could contribute to changes in VOR parameters. Smooth pursuit at high velocities and saccadic fixation of more peripheral targets does not mature until one year of age [Roucoux et al., 1983]. Thus, visual-vestibular interactions could differ in infants. One feature of visual-vestibular interaction is suppression of vestibular responses by visual fixation. We investigated the capacity of infants to suppress the VOR with visual fixation during low frequency sinusoidal stimulation. Also infant VOR characteristics (gain and phase) were assessed with impulsive and sinusoidal rotation for comparison with data on infants and adults previously obtained in our laboratories [Honrubia et al., 1984; Ornitz et al., 1985].

Methods

Thirteen infants (2–15 months old) and 10 adults received sinusoidal (60 deg/s, 0.0125 Hz) and impulsive (100 deg/s sudden velocity change) stimulation from rotation

Trial with fixation light

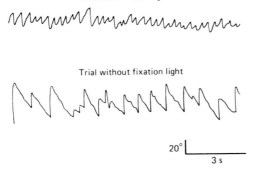

Trial without fixation light

20°

3 s

Fig. 1. Twelve-second samples of nystagmus during sinusoidal stimulation with and without fixation. Samples are taken close to time of maximum slow component velocity.

in complete darkness and sinusoidal stimulation with a head-fixed pinpoint red light in complete darkness. Horizontal eye movements were recorded from electrodes at the outer canthi on a polygraph, after DC amplification. The recording signal was calibrated, after dark adaptation, while the subject followed the instantaneous displacement of a fixation light (saccades in the correct direction within 0.6 s of light displacement).

The slow component velocity (SCV) of each nystagmus beat was measured from artifact-free segments of the polygraph records. The phase lead during sinusoidal stimulation was computed from the time of change of direction of the nystagmus to that of platform rotation. The time constant (TC) associated with this phase lead was computed from the relationship $TC = \tan(90° - phase lead)/2\pi f$. The time constant of nystagmus decay following impulse stimulation was computed as the time required for SCV to decrease to 37% of any previous velocity, using the slope of the least square regression line describing the relationship between the logarithm of the SCV and time after the impulse. Gains were expressed as the ratio of maximum SCV to maximum platform velocity.

All 13 infants provided data of sufficient quality to compute gains and TC in response to impulse stimulation. Because of movement, fussiness or sleepiness, adequate data could be obtained from only 8 of these 13 infants during sinusoidal stimulation without fixation and from 8 during sinusoidal stimulation with fixation. Infant and adult gains and TC were compared using two-sample t-tests (two-tailed).

Results

In all subjects, responses to sinusoidal stimulation with visual fixation showed nystagmus with smaller amplitudes and greater frequency (fig. 1, upper panel) than during trials without visual fixation (fig. 1, lower panel). This demonstrated that the infants did attend to and fixate the head-fixed target light. However, they showed a weak suppression of VOR gain during fixation. In the infants, VOR gain during fixation trials was 0.46 ± 0.15 while adults showed complete gain suppression (p <0.01).

During sinusoidal stimulation in the dark without fixation, the gains were significantly greater in the infants (0.89 ± 0.33) than in the adults (0.41 ± 0.12) (p <0.01). During impulsive stimulation, the gains were also significantly greater in the infants (1.32 ± 0.31) than in the adults (0.59 ± 0.20 (p <0.01).

TC derived from phase angles were significantly shorter in the infants (11.4 ± 3.2 s) than the adults (18.1 ± 4.8 s) (p <0.01). There were no differences between the TC of the infants (10.8 ± 2.8 s) and adults (9.9 ± 3.4 s) in response to impulsive stimulation.

Discussion

An analysis of these data in the context of current models of VOR function indicates that infants have greater sensitivities and shorter TC than adults. Within the range of frequencies used in this study, the VOR responses are determined by three parameters, a sensitivity coefficient (G_v) and two TC, a shorter one (T_v) and a longer one (T_a), reflecting the visco-elastic and adaptive properties of the inner ear, and the influence upon them of central nervous system mechanisms. The transfer function (Tf) of the VOR is given in Laplace notation by the following equation:

$$Tf = [(G_v sT_v)/(1 + sT_v)] \, [(sT_a)/(1 + sT_a)].$$

Because the adaptation time constant has been difficult to evaluate, the second term of the transfer function has often been ignored when only an approximate solution in the interpretation of the data has been required and if the responses are in the range of normal head movements. In this case, the model predicts that during high frequency rotations (about 1.0 Hz) the gain of the VOR approximates G_v, thus providing a direct measurement of VOR sensitivity. Since impulsive angular accelerations behave similarly to high frequency stimuli, our data show that G_v in infants is 2.2 times greater than adults. The same conclusion is obtained when G_v is computed from the sinusoidal data at 0.0125 Hz: $G_v = $ gain $[1 + (2\pi f T_v)^2]^{1/2}/(2\pi f T_v)$. The infants' G_v is 1.34 while that of the adults is 0.50. The predominant TC of the VOR in adults (T_v) obtained using the simplified pendulum model is shorter when derived from impulsive than sinusoidal data, a difference that is due to the neglect of the contribution of the adaptation operator $[sT_a/(1 + sT_a)]$ in the computation of VOR dynamics. In the infants, unlike the adults, the value of T_v from impulsive data (10.8 s) is not significantly different from that of sinusoidal data (11.4 s), suggesting the minimal influence of adaptation.

What is the reason for the difference in T_v and G_v between infants and adults? The minimal visual-vestibular interaction effects in the infants and the well-known influence of visual experience on the VOR suggest that in infancy, visual experience is not yet sufficient to modulate VOR function. The larger amplitude of the fast component of the nystagmus and the failure of fixation suppression of the VOR might reflect this lack of visual experience and/or immaturity of connectivity involving cerebellar and brain stem mechanisms. These centers of vestibular modulation may not be mature enough to fine tune the VOR.

References

Honrubia, V.; Jenkins, H.A.; Baloh, R.W.; Yee, R.D.; Lau, C.G.Y.: Vestibulo-ocular reflexes in peripheral labyrinthine lesions. I, Unilateral dysfunction. Am. J. Otolaryngol. *5:* 15–26 (1984).

Jager, J.; Henn, V.: Vestibular habituation in man and monkey during sinusoidal rotation; in Cohen, Vestibular and oculomotor physiology. Int. Meet. Barany Society, vol. 374, p. 330 (New York Academy of Sciences, New York 1981).

Ornitz, E.M.: Development of the vestibular system; in Meisami, Timiras, Handbook of human growth and developmental biology, vol. I (in press).

Ornitz, E.M.; Kaplan, A.R.; Westlake, J.R.: Development of the vestibulo-ocular reflex from infancy to adulthood. Acta oto-lar. *100:* 180–193 (1985).

Roucoux, A.; Culee, C.; Roucoux, M.: Development of fixation and pursuit eye movements in human infants. Behav. Brain Res. *10:* 133–139 (1983).

Edward M. Ornitz, MD, Division of Mental Retardation and Child Psychiatry, Department of Psychiatry, UCLA School of Medicine, 760 Westwood Plaza, Los Angeles, CA 90024 (USA)

Adv. Oto-Rhino-Laryng., vol. 41, pp. 40–43 (Karger, Basel 1988)

High Frequency Rotation Test: Clinical and Research Application

Vijay S. Dayal[a], *Mabel Mai*[b], *R. David Tomlinson*[c]

[a]Otolaryngology-Head and Neck Surgery, University of Chicago, Chicago, Ill., USA;
[b]Otolaryngology, University of Toronto, [c] Playfair Neuroscience Unit,
University of Toronto, Toronto, Ont., Canada

This article reviews our experiences with high frequency rotation test and its application for clinical and research work in humans [Dayal et al., 1987a, b; Mai et al., 1986]. Healthy subjects under the influence of barbiturates and patients with established diagnosis of Ménière's disease form the basis of this review.

Normal subjects provide the baseline data; findings in subjects under the influence of barbiturates we believe reflect central changes; findings in patients with Ménière's disease are, of course, due to peripheral changes. These data for each category have been published before [Dayal et al, 1987a, b; Mai et al., 1986]. In this paper we compare the high frequency rotation test findings in these three groups.

Material and Methods

Details of tests and analysis have been published [Schwarz and Tomlinson, 1979; Tomlinson et al., 1980; Hyden et al., 1982; Dayal et al., 1987a, b; Mai et al., 1986]. There were 17 healthy subjects, 20 healthy subjects in whom the effect of barbiturates (100–150 mg) was assessed and 11 patients with an established diagnosis of Ménière's disease. In brief, high frequency pseudorandom stimulus in a range of 0.3–5 Hz (maximum velocity 110 deg/s) was used. Vestibulo-ocular reflex (VOR) gain and cancellation (VORC) were determined. In normal subjects and subjects under the influence of barbiturate, tests were carried out for measurement of horizontal smooth pursuit tracking and saccades.

Table I. Percentage differences in VOR gain from normative data at various frequencies

	Frequency, Hz														
	0.32	0.61	0.90	1.2	1.49	2.08	2.37	2.66	2.95	3.25	3.54	3.83	4.13	4.42	4.71
Ménière's group	−11	−8	+2	−2	0	0	+4	+6	+22	+22	+24	+12	+14	16	—
Barbiturate group: 1 h post-ingestion	−7	−12	−12	−11	−14	−15	−17	−19	−21	−20	−12	−16	−16	−13	−14
Barbiturate group: 3 h post-ingestion	−3	−7	−5	−6	−5	−5	−7	−10	−6	−8	+2	−2	−4	−3	−4

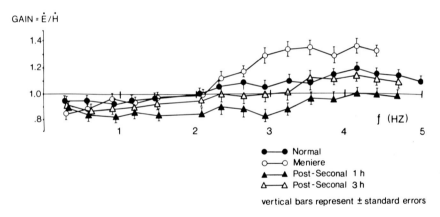

Fig. 1. Mean values of VOR gain at various frequencies.

Findings and Discussion

We will first discuss the clinical application followed by research application of high frequency vestibular testing in humans. The VOR gain and
VORC of the three groups are detailed in table I and shown in figure 1. The
normal subjects had a VOR gain of less than one up to about 2 Hz and a gain
slightly higher than one above that frequency. Similar gain above one has
been described by Benson [1970] in humans and Keller [1978] in monkeys.

Subjects under the influence of barbiturates show a very different picture. In the first hour post-ingestion, when blood levels are high, the VOR gain is below one up to approximately 4 Hz when it reaches a gain close to one. Three hours post-ingestion, when blood levels are lower compared to 1 h post-ingestion, the VOR gain is less than one up to approximately 3 Hz and then increases to more than one above this frequency. This is in sharp contrast to 1 h post-ingestion where the impairment of VOR gain was most pronounced. It is also in contrast to the VOR gain in normal subjects. As barbiturates act centrally it is reasonable to infer that the VOR gain reduction is a reflection of centrally induced change. The effects of barbiturates on the brain stem and cerebellum have been well documented [Bender and O'Brien, 1946; Norris, 1971; Haciska, 1973], and the drug achieves a high level in the CNS before being gradually distributed to other parts of the body [Harvey, 1980]. Patients with Ménière's disease on the other hand, show a slightly reduced gain compared to normals at the lowest test frequency. However, the VOR gain is similar to normal subjects up to 2 Hz when a gain of one is obtained. In the high frequencies, however, in these patients VOR shows a supranormal gain, reminiscent of cochlear recruitment in Ménière's disease [Fowler, 1937], an endorgan disease. This supranormal VOR gain in endorgan disease is in sharp contrast to the reduced VOR gain seen in centrally induced changes by barbiturates. These findings suggest that VOR testing at high frequencies may provide valuable information in the differential diagnosis of central and peripheral pathology and that further studies are indicated to explore this possibility.

The different types and degrees of changes seen in VOR gain with different levels of barbiturates suggest that high frequency vestibular test may be a useful tool in investigation of vestibulo-suppressive drugs. This is one possible research application of this test. As we have described before [Dayal et al., 1987 b; Mai et al., 1986], some basic physiological information in humans can be provided by high frequency vestibular stimulation combined with smooth pursuit testing. Briefly the time course of recovery of pursuit gain and VOR cancellation was dissimilar under the influence of barbiturates, providing further evidence that VOR cancellation and pursuit systems are subserved by different mechanisms [Robinson, 1982; Tomlinson and Robinson, 1980; Chambers and Gresty, 1983]. Similar studies with centrally acting pharmacological agents have the potential to provide valuable information not only about the physiology in humans but also about pathology in humans, albeit pharmacologically induced central changes.

References

Bender, M.B.; O'Brien, A.H.: The influence of barbiturate on various forms of nystagmus. Am. J. Ophthal. *29:* 1541 (1946).

Benson, A.J.: Interactions between semicircular canals and gravireceptors; in Busby, Recent advances in aerospace medicine, pp. 249–261 (Reidel Publishing, Dotrecht 1970).

Chambers, B.R.; Gresty, M.A.: The relationship between disordered pursuit and vestibulo-ocular reflex suppression. J. Neurol. Neurosurg. Psychiat. *46:* 61 (1983).

Dayal, V.S.; Mai, M.; Tomlinson, R.D.: Diagnostic abnormalities of high frequency rotation test in patients with Meniere's disease. Proc. Annu. Meet. of American Neurotology Society, Denver, 1987a.

Dayal, V.S.; Mai, M.; Tomlinson, R.D.; Farkashidy, J.: Effects of barbiturate on the vestibular and oculomotor systems. A sequential study; in The vestibular system — neurophysiologic and clinical research (Raven Press, New York, in press, 1987b).

Fowler, E.P.: The diagnosis of diseases of the neural mechanisms of hearing by the aid of sounds well above threshold. Laryngoscope *47:* 289 (1937).

Haciska, D.T.: The influence of drugs on caloric-induced nystagmus. Acta oto-lar. *75:* 477 (1973).

Harvey, S.C.: Hypnotics and sedatives; in Gilman, Goodman, Gilman, The pharmacological basis of therapeutics; 6th ed., p. 339 (Macmillan, New York 1980).

Hyden, D.; Istl, T.E.; Schwarz, D.W.F.: Human visuo-vestibular interaction as a basis for quantitative clinical diagnostics. Acta otolaryngol. *94:* 53 (1982).

Keller, E.L.: Gain of the vestibulo-ocular reflex in monkeys at high rotational frequencies. Vision Res. *18:* 311 (1978).

Mai, M.; Dayal, V.S.; Tomlinson, R.D.; Farkashidy, J.: Study of pursuit and vestibulo-ocular cancellation. Otolaryngol. Head Neck Surg, *95:* 589 (1986).

Norris, H.: The action of sedatives on brainstem oculomotor systems in man. Neuropharmacology *10:* 181 (1971).

Robinson, D.A.: A model of cancellation of the vestibulo-ocular reflex; in Lennerstrand, Zee, Keller, Functional basis of ocular motility disorders. (Pergamon Press, Oxford 1982).

Schwarz, D.W.F.; Tomlinson, R.D.: Diagnostic precision in a new rotatory vestibular test. J. Otolaryngol. *8:* 544 (1979).

Tomlinson, R.D.; Robinson, D.A.: Response of vestibular nuclei cells during vertical vestibular and pursuit eye movements. Soc. Neurosci. Abstr. *6:* 477 (1980).

Tomlinson, R.D.; Saunders, G.E.; Schwarz, D.W.F.: Analysis of human vestibulo-ocular reflex during active head movements. Acta oto-lar. *90:* 184–190 (1980).

Dr. V.S. Dayal, Otolaryngology-Head and Neck Surgery, University of Chicago Medical Center, Box 412, 5841 South Maryland Avenue, Chicago, IL 60637 (USA)

Adv. Oto-Rhino-Laryng., vol. 41, pp. 44–48 (Karger, Basel 1988)

Impaired Discharge of the Eye Velocity Storage Mechanism in Patients with Lesions of the Vestibulo-Cerebellum

W. Heide, V. Schrader, E. Koenig, J. Dichgans

Department of Neurology, University of Tübingen, Tübingen, FRG

Introduction

The slower decline of postrotatory nystagmus ($\tau = 10–20$ s) as compared to the modulation of the discharge rate of peripheral vestibular afferents ($\tau = 5–8$ s) has been attributed to an eye velocity storage mechanism [Raphan et al., 1979], presumably located in or near the vestibular nuclei. The time constant (τ) of postrotatory nystagmus ($= PI$) is markedly shortened after short periods of visual fixation of a subject-stationary single target or full-field surround [Raphan et al., 1979; Koenig and Dichgans, 1981; Waespe and Schwarz, 1986] or with passive or active changes of head position from the prior upright position in relation to gravity [Benson and Bodin, 1966; Raphan et al., 1981; Schrader et al., 1985]. This phenomenon has been termed 'dumping', according to the assumption that it is due to a rapid discharge of the velocity storage mechanism, induced both by head tilt (most probably mediated by the otoliths) and visual fixation. Since recent monkey experiments [Waespe et al., 1985] have shown that the dumping is lost after ablation of the cerebellar nodulus and uvula, we investigated whether analogous findings in cerebellar patients can be used for functional testing of the inferior vermis in humans.

Methods

Four patients (aged 33–66 years) with cerebellar lesions around the midline, mainly of the vestibulo-cerebellum (one case after surgery of a dermoid in vermis and nodulus as

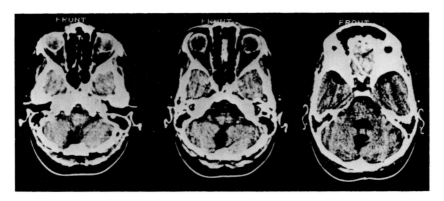

Fig. 1. CAT scan of a 34-year-old female who underwent surgery of a dermoid in cerebellar vermis and nodulus 3 years ago.

shown in figure 1, one case of Arnold-Chiari malformation, one case of cavernous angioma extending caudally from the 4th ventricle near the midline and one case of cerebellar atrophy with downbeat nystagmus) were tested in comparison to a control group of normals (5 subjects aged 25–60 years). Oculomotor abnormalities in the patients were square wave jerks, saccadic dysmetria, gaze nystagmus, rebound nystagmus and slight impairments of smooth pursuit, optokinetic nystagmus and fixation suppression of vestibulo-ocular reflex (VOR) in all 4 cases. Hyperexcitability of VOR was present in 3 cases, downbeat nystagmus in one patient and positional downbeat nystagmus in another patient.

Eye movements were recorded by DC electro-oculography. Subjects were accelerated at a rate of 18 °/s^2 for 10 s in darkness. After reaching the maximum velocity of 180 °/s, a subject-stationary full-field surround was presented for 5 s, during which the subjects had to fixate. Again in darkness, the residual perrotatory nystagmus was recorded. In a second experiment, the chair was suddenly stopped; 4 s after the stop, subjects were asked to bend their heads 90° forward. This experiment was performed in both directions and — as control — also without visual fixation and head tilt.

Results

Table I shows the cumulative amplitudes of perrotatory and postrotatory nystagmus of normals (NP) and patients (CP), both with and without visual fixation and head tilt. Whereas the average cumulative amplitude was reduced by 59% after visual fixation in normals, it remained the same in patients. Forward head tilt led to a much stronger reduction of cumulative amplitude in normals (−71%) than in patients (−14%). The vestibular excitability in control trials (without fixation and head tilt) showed no clear

Table I. Cumulative amplitude (degrees)

	5 s visual fixation		90 ° head tilt forward	
	without	with	without	with
NP	334	137	979	284
CP	294	293	856	735

Table II. Time constant (seconds)

	5 s visual fixation		90 ° head tilt forward	
	without	with	without	with
NP	10.8	8.9	13.7	5.8
CP	10.0	10.4	10.3	7.7

difference between normals and patients. The obviously higher cumulative amplitude with head tilt as compared to visual fixation results from the fact that in the former, the computation included the complete postrotatory nystagmus, whereas in the latter, perrotatory nystagmus was only included after the fixation interval. Time constants as determined by a single exponential showed similar results (table II) with a reduction of 14% after visual fixation and 58% after head tilt for normals, whereas patients again showed no (visual fixation) or only a minor reduction (by 25% with head tilt).

As an example, in figure 2 the velocity profile of perrotatory nystagmus with and without visual fixation (the fixation interval of 5 s is indicated on the abscissa) is plotted for the patient whose CAT scan is shown in figure 1. There is a reduction of nystagmus velocity during the presentation of the stationary surround and its attempted fixation. Again in darkness, nystagmus velocity jumps back to the level of perrotatory nystagmus without fixation. Also the further decline is almost identical so that there is no indication for a discharge of the velocity storage mechanism by fixation.

Figure 3 shows a comparison of the velocity profiles of the same patient's postrotatory nystagmus with and without head tilt, with a virtually identical decline of nystagmus velocity, i.e. again a missing discharge of the velocity storage.

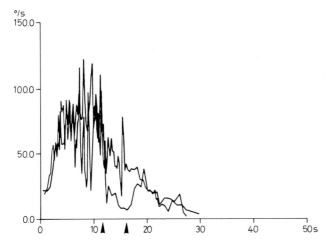

Fig. 2. Slow phase velocity profiles of perrotatory nystagmus (caused by acceleration of 18 °/s^2 during the first 10 s) with and without 5 s of visual fixation, shown for the case of figure 1. The fixation interval is indicated on the abscissa.

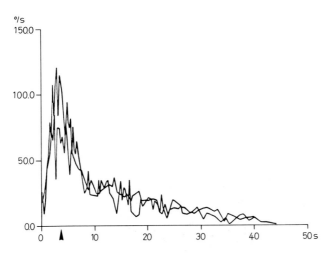

Fig. 3. Slow phase velocity profiles of postrotatory nystagmus with and without 90° head tilt forward, 4 s after stop out of 180 °/s constant velocity rotation in darkness, shown for the case of figure 1. The head tilt is indicated on the abscissa.

Conclusions

We conclude that the rapid discharge of the eye velocity storage mechanism caused by visual fixation or active head tilt is markedly impaired in patients with lesions of the cerebellar nodulus and neighboring structures. Amplitude and time constant of vestibular nystagmus remain unchanged after visual fixation and are only slightly reduced by active head tilt, which might be attributed to a possible direct inhibitory influence of the still intact otolith function. Our results correspond to those obtained by Waespe et al. [1985] in lesioned monkeys. The discharge of the velocity storage mechanism thus may turn out to be a specific test for inferior vermis function in clinical practice. Its specificity, however, remains to be seen, because other cerebellar oculomotor symptoms were present as well.

References

Benson, A.J.; Bodin, M.A.: Effect of orientation to gravitational vertical on nystagmus following rotation about a horizontal axis. Acta oto-lar. 61: 517–526 (1966).
Koenig, E.; Dichgans, J.: Aftereffects of vestibular and optokinetic stimulation. Ann. N.Y. Acad. Sci. 374: 434–445 (1981).
Raphan, T.; Cohen, B.; Henn, V.: Effects of gravity on rotatory nystagmus in monkeys. Ann. N.Y. Acad. Sci. 374: 44–55 (1981).
Raphan, T.; Matsuo, V.; Cohen, B.: Velocity storage in the vestibulo-ocular reflex arc (VOR). Exp. Brain Res. 35: 229–238 (1979).
Schrader, V.; Koenig, E.; Dichgans, J.: Direction and angle of active head tilts influencing the Purkinje effect and the inhibition of postrotatory nystagmus I and II. Acta otolaryngol 100: 337–343 (1985).
Waespe, W.; Cohen, B.; Raphan, T.: Dynamic modification of the vestibulo-ocular reflex by the nodulus and uvula. Science 228: 199–202 (1985).
Waespe, W.; Schwarz, U.: Characteristics of eye velocity storage during periods of suppression and reversal of eye velocity in monkeys. Exp. Brain Res. 65: 49–58 (1986).

W. Heide, MD, Department of Neurology, University of Tübingen,
D-7400 Tübingen (FRG)

Adv. Oto-Rhino-Laryng., vol. 41, pp. 49–52 (Karger, Basel 1988)

Vertical Canal Stimulation Abolishes Horizontal Velocity Storage: Effects on Optokinetic Nystagmus and Eye Movements Evoked by a Rotating Linear Acceleration

Laurence R. Harris

Department of Physiology, University College, Cardiff, UK

For clear vision a stable retinal image is required. During head movements the eyes make compensatory rotations which tend to cancel movements of the retinal image. Head movements are detected by several mechanisms that contribute to this response. The mechanisms of the canal- and visual-evoked (optokinetic nystagmus, OKN) responses share a stored neural representation of the velocity of the head movement which acts like a flywheel and usefully prolongs the response beyond the duration of the stimulus [1–3].

Whenever the axis of a rotatory head movement is not perfectly vertical, the pattern of the stimulation of the otoliths (which detect linear accelerations: here gravity) conveys information about the continually changing direction of tilt during the rotation [4, 5]. A constant-velocity off-vertical-axis rotation (OVAR) is accompanied by a continuous compensatory nystagmus [4, 5] (fig. 2a) in the cat. If the animal is rotated until the canal-evoked response has decayed and then the axis tilted, compensatory eye movements build up with a time constant of about 5 s [5, 6]. This suggests the charging of a velocity store which may be held in common.

Stimulating the vertical canals by sudden tilting during optokinetic afternystagmus (OKAN) suddenly discharges the visually charged velocity store [4]. OKN and OKAN (which depend on an intact velocity store [1, 2, 7]) were therefore measured during continuous sinusoidal activation of the vertical canals. Figure 1 contrasts OKN evoked in a stationary animal with that

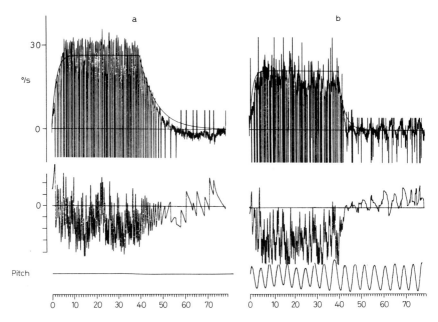

Fig. 1. OKN in response to horizontal, full-field, visual movement produced by a planetarium projector projecting spots onto a 57-cm radius spherical screen centred on the cat's head. Eye movements were recorded from 3 cats with implanted scleral search coils. The animals were held at the centre of the screen by head restraining tubes (Kopf). The stimulus was moving at 30 °/s. The traces represent, from the top, horizontal eye velocity, horizontal eye position and pitch. The lights went out after 40 s. *a* Stimulation around a stationary vertical axis. Note the gradual decline of OKAN (time constant 7.4 s). The line through the data was derived from Robinson's model of velocity storage (K, the efficiency of the store = 0.65 [7], open-loop gain = 2.3 [8]). *b* The response to exactly the same optokinetic stimulus as in *a*, but in this case with simultaneous pitch of ± 20° at 0.23 Hz. The line plotted through the data has again been derived from Robinson's [7] model (K = 0).

obtained with exactly the same visual stimulus during simultaneous sinusoidal pitch. The data suggest that pitching deactivates the horizontal velocity store. OKN and OKAN were measured in 3 cats during pitching movements (± 10 and ± 45°, 0.05–0.3 Hz). The gain (eye velocity/stimulus velocity) of OKN was attenuated to 0.7 ± 0.1 from its control values (0.94 ± 0.06) and the time constant of OKAN was reduced from 7.4 ± 2.8 to 1.5 ± 0.5 s.

In order to produce a rotating gravity vector with simultaneous stimulation of the vertical canals (and thus a deactivated velocity store), I subjected

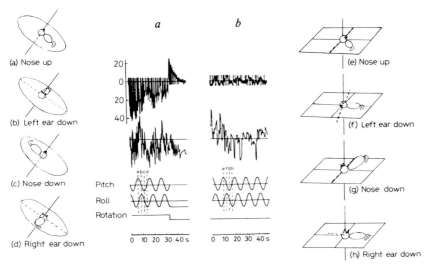

Fig. 2. Eye movements evoked by rotating linear accelerations in complete darkness. The traces represent, from the top: horizontal eye velocity and horizontal eye position, pitch (with respect to gravity: up represents up), roll (with respect to gravity: up represents left ear down), horizontal angular velocity (up represents leftward movement). *a* OVAR at 36 °/s to the left around an axis tilted at 20°. The initial canal response declines to a continuous, sinusoidally modulated nystagmus with an average velocity of 13 °/s. *b* The response to sequential tilting. The animal was rocked sinusoidally in the pitch and roll planes with a 90° phase difference as shown in the stimulus traces. This thus produced exactly the same pattern of stimulation of the otoliths as in *a*. It is equivalent to leftward rotation.

3 cats to 'sequential tilting' (fig. 2b). Although the changing tilt is the same in both OVAR and sequential tilting, the vertical canals are only stimulated during sequential tilt. In response to sequential tilting there is no horizontal nystagmus at all (fig. 2b). Sequential tilting was carried out in 3 cats (± 10–20°, 0.05–0.2 Hz: equivalent to OVAR of 18–72 °/s). In no case was any horizontal nystagmus evoked.

These data argue strongly for the involvement of a central velocity storage mechanism in the generation of the response to OVAR. Since OKN and OKAN are also affected (fig. 1) it further suggests that the velocity store that is involved in OVAR is also used by OKN (known to be shared by VOR) [1, 2]. Since the response to a rotating gravity vector is abolished completely, this suggests that there is no direct pathway in the system that processes OVAR.

References

1   Raphan, T.; Cohen, B.; Matsuo, V.: A velocity storage mechanism responsible for OKN, OKAN and vestibular nystagmus; in ref. [9].

2   Demer, J.L.; Robinson, D.A.: Different time constants for optokinetic and vestibular nystagmus with a single velocity storage element. Brain Res. *276:* 173–177 (1983).

3   Raphan, T.; Matsuo, V.; Cohen, B.: Velocity storage in the vestibulo-ocular reflex arc (VOR). Exp. Brain Res. *35:* 229–248 (1979).

4   Raphan, T.; Cohen, B.; Henn, V.: Effects of gravity on rotatory nystagmus in monkeys. Ann. N.Y. Acad. Sci. *374:* 44–55 (1981).

5   Harris, L.R.: Vestibular and optokinetic eye movements evoked in the cat by rotation about a tilted axis. Exp. Brain Res. *66:* 522–532 (1987).

6   Cohen, B.; Suzuki, J.; Raphan, T.; Matsuo, V.; Jong, V. de: Selective labyrinthine lesions and nystagmus induced by rotation about an off-vertical axis; in Lennerstrand, Keller, Zee, Functional basis of ocular motility disorders, pp. 337–346 (Pergamon, Oxford 1982).

7   Robinson, D.A.: Vestibular and optokinetic symbiosis: an example of explaining by modelling; in ref. [9].

8   Maioli, C.; Precht, W.: The horizontal optokinetic nystagmus in the cat. Exp. Brain Res. *55:* 494–506 (1984).

9   Baker, R.; Berthoz, A. (eds): Control of gaze by brain stem neurones (Elsevier/North-Holland, Amsterdam 1977).

Laurence R. Harris, PhD, Department of Physiology, University College, Cardiff CF1 1XL (UK)

Adv. Oto-Rhino-Laryng., vol. 41, pp. 53–57 (Karger, Basel 1988)

The Effect of Alertness on the Velocity Storage Mechanism

Måns Magnusson, Ilmari Pyykkö, Lucyna Schalén, Håkan Enbom

Department of Otorhinolaryngology, University Hospital of Lund, Lund, Sweden

Introduction

Alertness affects the vestibulo-ocular reflex (VOR) [1] and subcortically mediated optokinetic nystagmus (OKN) in man and animal [2, 3]. It is not well understood by what means alertness affects these oculo-motor reflexes. Both the VOR and subcortically mediated OKN converge on the so-called velocity storage mechanism in the central vestibular pathways [4, 5]. This functionally defined mechanism prolongs the short time constant of the vestibular nerve to the observed longer time constant of postrotatory nystagmus. When the visual image moves across the retina in optokinetic stimulation, the retinal slip, i.e. the difference between eye and image motion, will gradually charge the velocity storage mechanism which results in the slow rise of the velocity of slow phases of nystagmus typical for subcortically mediated OKN [6]. The response of subcortical OKN is concealed in foveate animals such as primates and man by the faster reacting cortical optokinetic pathway. In non-foveated animals, such as the rabbit, which lack the cortical pathways [7], the slow rise of the subcortical OKN can be observed.

When assessing a behavioral variable like alertness, it is important to use a stimulus which induces changes in the variable which can be ascertained both by behavioral correlates and neuro-physiologic measurements [8]. Rabbits exposed to vibration to the abdomen show both behavioral signs and exhibit characteristic patterns of increased alertness in intracerebral electro-encephalographic recordings [7].

The aim of the present study was to investigate if changes in the state of alertness affect the velocity storage mechanism, using rabbits in an experimental model.

Material and Methods

Eye movements were recorded with DC-electro-oculographic technique using implanted silver-silver chloride electrodes in 9 pigmented rabbits and printed out by an ink-jet writer. VOR were tested as postrotatory nystagmus evoked by velocity steps of 20, 40, 60, 90 and 120 °/s. Subcortical OKN was tested as the nystagmus response to whole field optokinetic stimulation, provided by a rotating striped drum surrounding the rabbit. Velocity steps of 10, 20, 30 and 40 °/s were used [9].

Minimum and maximum points of each slow phase were visually identified and fed into a UNIVAC host computer by plotting on an X—Y coordinate table. Slow phase velocities, time constants and gain were subsequently calculated by the computer. Calibration of the recordings was achieved by rotating the rabbits at 60 °/s in a lighted surrounding approximating the initial gain to 1.0. Calibration was then corrected using infrared video recording of a close-up view of the eye of the rabbit and the simultaneous ink-jet recording when the rabbit was rotated in darkness. Calculations on a split-screen video display allowed the ink-jet recorder to be calibrated for the absolute angle of eye deviation. The time constant of VOR was defined as the time needed for the decay of postrotatory nystagmus to reach $1/e$ of the initial gain. The time constant of OKN was defined as the time needed to reach $1-(1/e)$ of the steady-state velocity. Vibration of 125 Hz and 2.2-mm amplitude was used as alerting stimulus [9]. Student's t-test for paired data, in second-stage statistics [9], was used for evaluations.

Results

When rabbits were exposed to vibration during postrotatory nystagmus (fig. 1) the time constant of the VOR was significantly prolonged ($p < 0.001$), while the gain of VOR was not affected ($p <$n.s.).

The slow rise of OKN was significantly shorter (fig. 2) in the alerted than in the non-alerted rabbit ($p < 0.001$) while the steady-state gain remained unchanged.

Discussion

Increased alertness affects the VOR by prolonging the time constant and subcortical OKN by shortening the slow rise of OKN, whereas gain remains unchanged in both cases. The velocity storage mechanism is an observed function of the central vestibular pathway which 'stores' activity evoked by vestibular or optokinetic stimulation. This mechanism has been described as an 'imperfect or leaking integrator' [5] where the 'leak' corresponded to the magnitude of the central time constant of the velocity

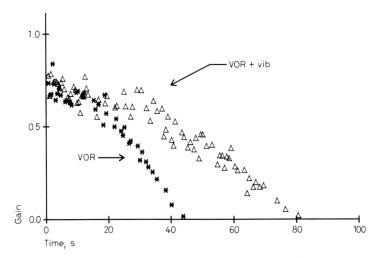

Fig. 1. Gain of slow phase velocity of postrotatory nystagmus in response to a 60 °/s velocity step in the same rabbit. Triangles denote response when the rabbit was alerted with vibration, stars when not.

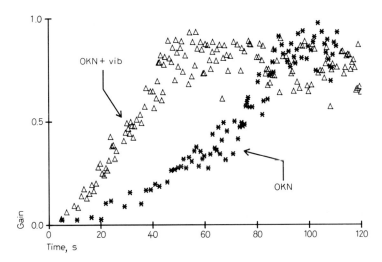

Fig. 2. Gain of slow phase velocity of OKN in response to a 30 °/s velocity step in the same rabbit. Triangles denote response when the rabbit was alerted with vibration, stars when not.

storage mechanism. Thus, the greater the 'leak' the shorter is the time constant.

The decay of slow phase velocity in the postrotatory nystagmus and the slow rise in subcortical OKN are controlled by the time constant of the same velocity storage mechanism [5]. Additionally, in the present study we found that changes of alertness change the time constants of VOR and subcortical OKN without affecting the gain. Thus, the present findings can be explained by alertness prolonging the central time constant of the velocity storage mechanism or, metaphorically, reducing 'the leak of the imperfect integrator'.

The use of the term 'time constant' in rabbits may be discussed since the decay of postrotatory nystagmus in rabbits is linear rather than exponential [9, 10]. Although the most accepted method of estimating the decay or increase of slow phase velocity has been the one used in the present study, other methods are possible. The decay or increase of slow phase velocity could be estimated by integrating the slow phase velocities over time defining the rise time to the point on the x-axis crossed by an asymptote of the steady-state velocity level or as the area under or over a fitted curve [for details, see refs. 4, 6]. Calculating the response by the latter methods did not, however, change the significance of our results. Thus, we have chosen the present method of estimating the decay or slow rise of slow phase velocity, being the most commonly employed.

References

1 Collins, W.E.: Arousal and vestibular habituation; in Kornhuber, Handbook of sensory physiology, vol. VI, part 2, pp. 361–368 (Springer, New York 1974).
2 Pyykkö, I.; Magnusson, M.: Neural activity, alertness and visual orientation in intact and unilaterally labyrinthectomized rabbits. ORL *49:* 26–35 (1987).
3 Magnusson, M.; Pyykkö, I.; Jäntti, V.: The effect of alertness and attention on optokinetic nystagmus in man. Am. J. Otolaryngol. *6:* 419–425 (1985).
4 Raphan, T.; Matsuo, V.; Cohen, B.: Velocity storage in the vestibulo-ocular reflex arc (VOR). Exp. Brain Res. *35:* 229–248 (1979).
5 Demer, J.L.; Robinson, D.A.: Different time constants for optokinetic and vestibular nystagmus with a single velocity-storage element. Brain Res. *276:* 173–177 (1983).
6 Cohen, B.; Matsuo, V.; Raphan, T.: Quantitative analysis of optokinetic nystagmus and optokinetic after nystagmus. J.. Physiol. *270:* 321–344 (1977).
7 Collewijn, H.: Integration of adaptive changes of the optokinetic reflex, pursuit and the vestibulo-ocular reflex; in Berthoz, Melville Jones, Adaptive mechanisms in gaze control. Facts and theories, pp. 51–69 (Elsevier, Amsterdam 1985).

8   Koella, W.P.: Vigilance—local vigilance—the vigilance profile: a new concept and its application in neurobiology and biological psychiatry. Acta neurol. scand. *69:* suppl. 99, pp. 35–41 (1984).

9   Magnusson, M.: Effect of alertness on the vestibulo-ocular reflex and on the slow rise in optokinetic nystagmus in rabbits. Am. J. Otolaryngol. *7:* 353–359 (1986).

10 Collewijn, H.; Winterson, B.J.; Steen, J. van der: Post-rotatory nystagmus and optokinetic after-nystagmus in the rabbit linear rather than exponential decay. Exp. Brain Res. *40:* 330–338 (1980).

Måns Magnusson, MD, Department of Otorhinolaryngology,
University Hospital of Lund, S-221 85 Lund (Sweden)

Adv. Oto-Rhino-Laryng., vol. 41, pp. 58–62 (Karger, Basel 1988)

Effect of VOR Gain Changes on OKR Gain Control in Human Subjects

Hideharu Aoki, Toshiaki Yagi

Department of Otolaryngology, Nippon Medical School, Bunkyo-ku, Tokyo, Japan

Introduction

The vestibulo-ocular reflex (VOR) helps maintain a stable retinal image by generating the appropriate compensatory eye movements. Recent observations in human subjects and animals [4, 6] have clearly established that VOR is plastic and adaptive in nature. On the other hand, the optokinetic system also serves to stabilize moving images on the retina. Under natural conditions, head movement produces relative movement of the surroundings and results in simultaneous stimulation of both vestibular and optokinetic systems. In this way, the VOR and optokinetic response (OKR) help to cooperatively stabilize retinal images.

Recent investigations [4–6] have shown that the visual and vestibular inputs are integrated in the vestibular nucleus. Lisberger et al. [3] and Robinson [6] reported that in animals the vestibular nucleus neurons respond to both vestibular and optokinetic inputs. This result suggests that the elements responsible for the VOR gain changes are in a part of the vestibulo-ocular pathway that is shared with the optokinetic system. The adaptive increases or decreases in VOR gain may thus cause parallel changes in the OKR gain. In fact, recent examinations in cats [2] and monkeys [3] have shown that the VOR gain changes indeed affect the OKR gain.

We previously reported [1] that in human subjects wearing vision reversal prisms, the gain control of the VOR and OKR was not independent. In other words, the reduction of the VOR gain by vision reversal prisms caused a decrease in the OKR gain. Our recent concern, however, has been that magnifying spectacles might affect both the VOR and OKR gain control in opposition to the vision reversal prisms. The principal aim of the present study was to investigate the effects of magnified vision on the adaptive changes of the VOR and OKR gains in human subjects.

Method

Ten normal adult subjects who were free from vestibular and oculomotor disorders, ranging in age from 24 to 39 years, were employed in this study. Their horizontal OKR were examined in a full-field optokinetic drum incorporating stripes at constant angular velocities of 30, 60, 90, and 120 °/s. The VOR gains in the dark were then examined under horizontal pendular rotation at a 0.25 Hz frequency and a 30° angular amplitude. Slow phase eye velocities of the OKR and VOR gains in the dark were measured by electro-oculography (EOG).

The VOR gain is defined as the eye velocity divided by the head velocity. Accordingly, we adopted a relative VOR gain, which was defined as the eye velocity in the dark divided by eye velocity under gazing conditions, because it is nearly equal to the head velocity at this relatively low-frequency range of pendular rotation. The OKR gain is defined as slow phase eye velocity, which is calculated from EOG, divided by the drum velocity.

Each subject was subsequently asked to wear magnifying spectacles ($\times$2) and was rotated on a chair sinusoidally for 1 h for the purpose of forced adaptation. After removing the spectacles, the VOR and OKR gains were examined again in a similar way.

Results

The VOR gain in the dark was found to be increased from 0.47 ± 0.09 to 0.62 ± 0.08 after wearing the magnifying spectacles for 1 h. These values differ significantly ($p < 0.01$; two-tailed t-test). The means and standard deviations of the slow phase eye velocity of OKR before wearing spectacles at 30, 60, 90 and 120 °/s were 29.3 ± 3.2, 58.1 ± 6.4, 82.4 ± 10.8 and 96.1 ± 22.0, respectively. After wearing the spectacles for the time period, these values changed to 27.9 ± 3.2, 53.9 ± 7.5, 76.9 ± 13.1 and 86.5 ± 16.2 (fig. 1), respectively. The means and standard deviations of the OKR gains at 30, 60, 90 and 120 °/s before wearing the spectacles were 0.98 ± 0.11, 0.97 ± 0.11, 0.91 ± 0.12 and 0.80 ± 0.18, respectively. After the spectacles were worn for the experimental period, the OKR gains at the same stimulus speeds were 0.93 ± 0.11, 0.90 ± 0.13, 0.85 ± 0.14 and 0.72 ± 0.14 (fig. 2), respectively. Importantly, no statistically significant differences were noted in the OKR gain before and after wearing magnifying spectacles at any drum velocity.

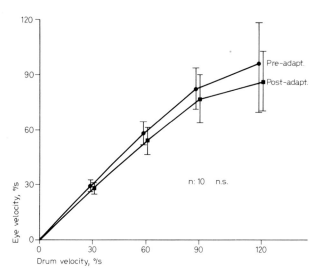

Fig. 1. Slow phase eye velocity of OKR before and after VOR adaptation produced by magnifying spectacles. Filled circles and squares indicate means of slow phase eye velocity of OKR before and after wearing spectacles, respectively. Vertical bars indicate standard deviations.

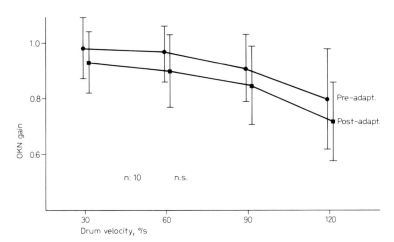

Fig. 2. OKR gains before and after VOR adaptation produced by magnifying spectacles.

Discussion

We previously reported [1] that the VOR gain was significantly reduced from 0.59 to 0.37 under the conditions of employing vision reversal prisms along with pendular rotation for 1 h. We also indicated that the OKR gain before and after wearing vision reversal prisms was significantly reduced 12–19% with each drum velocity value. The result obtained under VOR adaptation, derived from vision reversal prisms, indicates that the variable gain element affected by the wearing of vision reversal prisms is common to both VOR and optokinetic systems. In other words, the VOR and OKR gain control systems are not independent, and each response shared a common gain element in human subjects as well as in other animals [2, 3].

Our recent concern, however, has been that magnifying spectacles might affect both the VOR and OKR gain control in opposition to the vision reversal prisms. Under the present experimental conditions, however, the adaptive increased VOR gain produced by the magnifying spectacles indicated no effect on the OKR gain control in human subjects. This result differs from the results reported in other animals [2, 3], where the adaptively increased VOR gain produced by magnifying spectacles caused the increase in the OKR gains. The reason for this difference, however, is not clear.

Demer [2] reported in his cat experiment that regardless of the VOR gain values, most cats were able to closely match the drum velocity up to 20 °/s. The higher the drum velocity, however, the VOR gain changes were shown to affect the VOR gain values. Lisberger et al. [3] also reported that with monkeys a relationship of the gains between OKR and VOR was most evident for a low VOR gain or higher drum velocity. These experiments suggest that the adaptive VOR gain changes toward the decrease produces a greater effect on the OKR gain than does the increase. The effect of VOR gain changes on OKR gain control appears in higher optokinetic stimulation than in lower stimulation. Thus, we speculate that the velocity range of the optokinetic stimuli used in the present study is insufficient to detect the OKR gain changes which may be produced by the VOR gain changes induced by the magnifying spectacles in human subjects.

Conclusion

In human subjects, the adaptive change of the VOR gain, which is induced by vision reversal prisms, produces parallel changes on the OKR gain as it does as well in other animals. Under the present experimental conditions, however, the adaptively increased VOR gain generated by magnifying spectacles indicated no effect on the OKR gain control.

References

1   Aoki, H.; Yagi, T.; Kobayashi, Y.; Kamio, T.: Effect of VOR gain changes on OKR gain control; in Graham, Barany Society Proc., Ann Arbor (Raven Press, New York 1987).
2   Demer, J.L.: The variable gain element of the vestibulo-ocular reflex is common to the optokinetic system of the cat. Brain Res. *229:* 1–13 (1981).
3   Lisberger, S.G.; Miles, F.A.; Optican, L.M.; Eighmy, B.B.: Optokinetic response in monkey: underlying mechanisms and their sensitivity to long-term adaptive changes in vestibulo-ocular reflex. J. Neurophysiol. *45:* 869–890 (1981).
4   Miles, F.A.; Lisberger, S.G.: Plasticity in the vestibulo-ocular reflex: a new hypothesis. A. Rev. Neurosci. *4:* 273–299 (1984).
5   Precht, W.; Strata, P.: On the pathway mediating optokinetic response in vestibular nucleus neurons. Neuroscience *5:* 777–778 (1980).
6   Robinson, D.A.: Adaptive gain control of vestibulo-ocular reflex by cerebellum. J. Neurophysiol. *39:* 954–969 (1976).

Hideharu Aoki, MD, Department of Otolaryngology, Nippon Medical School, 1-1-5 Sendagi, Bunkyo-ku, Tokyo 113 (Japan)

Adv. Oto-Rhino-Laryng., vol. 41, pp. 63–70 (Karger, Basel 1988)

Visual Modulatory Influences of Vestibulo-Ocular Reflex in Patients with Vertigo[1]

K. Mizukoshi, H. Kobayashi, N. Ohashi, Y. Watanabe

Department of Otolaryngology, Toyama Medical and Pharmaceutical University, Toyama City, Japan

Introduction

The posture and body equilibrium mechanism is regulated by multisensory modalities from visual, vestibular and proprioceptive systems. However, there are few observations on the multisensory modalities of the equilibrium system in patients with vertigo [2, 8, 9].

On the other hand, many clinical observations have been made on harmonic sinusoidal rotation tests using a torque motor-driven system with mini-computer analysis [1]. Therefore, in order to readily detect abnormal visual influence of vestibulo-ocular reflex (VOR), we first investigated the visual vestibulo-ocular (V-VOR) gains in pendular rotation with eyes open in a stationary optokinetic (OK) drum, and then the fixation suppression in caloric nystagmus in normal subjects and in patients with vertigo.

Test Subjects

Of 133 patients with peripheral vestibular disorders, 49 had definite Ménière's disease, 46 had sudden deafness with vertigo and/or dizziness and 38 had benign paroxysmal positional vertigo (BPPV). On the other hand, out of 94 patients with CNS lesions 23 had cerebellar lesions, 34 had brain stem lesions, 26 had combined brain stem cerebellar lesions and 8 had cerebellopontine angle lesions. In each case, the history and neurotological findings conformed with neurotological diagnosis, and the locations of the definite lesions were also confirmed by surgical or radiological documentation.

[1] This work was supported in part by Grant 60570807 from the Ministry of Education of Japan

Electronystagmography and Analysis System

Eye movements were recorded by means of ENG with a time constant of 4.0 s or with DC recording. Paper speed was 3 or 5 mm/s. Arousal was maintained by mental arithmetic. The data was digitized at 100–200 samples per second and was analyzed with PDP 11/34 computer system with the aid of programs which were written in Assembler language by Watanabe et al. [11]. Each slow-phase velocity of the OKN, VOR and V-VOR and caloric nystagmus tests was plotted on the X-Y plotter. However, the phase-lags were not evaluated in this observation.

Test Procedure

The test subjects were rotated sinusoidally in the center of the OK drum. For pendular OKN testing, the test subjects were instructed not to follow the sinusoidally rotating stripes, but rather to count them during the pendular OK drum test. Then, for VOR testing, patients were rotated sinusoidally in the center of a dark OK drum, and finally were instructed to open their eyes in the illuminated OK drum. In the V-VOR testing, they were also instructed to count the stripes. In this test battery the OK stripes and the chair were rotated for the same period of 10 s and with the same amplitude of 120° (peak velocity: 75.4°/s). During this test battery, the OKN, VOR and V-VOR gains in the maximum slow-phase velocities were measured for three cycles with eyes open and three more with eyes closed and finally for three more with eyes open in an illuminated OK drum.

For fixation suppression testing, the test subjects were requested to keep their eyes open and fixed on one point for 10–55 s after the onset of air or water irrigation. They were then asked to close their eyes for the next 10 s to do mental arithmetic. Details of the caloric pattern test and calculation of percentage reduction in slow-phase velocity were reported by Kato et al. [3].

According to our experimental and clinical studies, cases with less than a 50% reduction induced by fixation were referred to as failure of fixation suppression (i.e. FFS) in caloric responses.

Results and Comments

Normal Limits of the OKN, VOR and V-VOR Tests

By means of PDP 11/34 computer analysis, normal limits of the OKN, VOR and V-VOR tests were calculated for the nystagmus responses in the 34 normal subjects during sinusoidal stimulation. From these normal values of the OKN, VOR and V-VOR gains, the normal limits of DP% were also calculated for clinical practice, as shown in table I. The calculation was made in accordance with the formula set up by Wolfe et al. [12].

Table I. Normal limits in the P-OKN, VOR and V-VOR tests

Condition	Gain (mean $\pm$ SD)	DP, %
P-OKN (eyes open)	0.88 $\pm$ 0.15	10
VOR (eyes closed)	0.76 $\pm$ 0.19	10
V-VOR (eyes open)	0.93 $\pm$ 0.13	5

Amplitude, 120°; frequency, 0.1 Hz; n = 34.

Table II. Abnormal VOR and V-VOR gains in the 133 patients with peripheral vestibular disorders

Abnormal VOR and V-VOR gains	Ménière's disease (n = 49)[1]	Sudden deafness (n = 46)	BPPV (n = 38)
VOR-DP V-VOR (—)	24	16	5
VOR (—) V-VOR (—)	13	20	22
VOR ↓ V-VOR (—)	5	6	7
VOR ↓ V-VOR ↓	4	4	4

(—) = Normal; ↓ = decreased; ↑ = increased gains.
[1] Another 3 cases showed increased VOR gains with normal V-VOR gains.

Patients with Peripheral Vestibular Disorders

OKN, VOR and V-VOR Gains in the 133 Patients. Comparing the OKN, VOR and V-VOR gains in the patients with the three different diseases, VOR-DP with normal OKN and V-VOR gain were more frequently observed in patients with Ménière's disease (24 cases) and sudden deafness (16 cases) than in those with BPPV (5 cases) (table II). In all 7 patients with bilateral peripheral lesions, such as Ménière's disease (5 cases) and sudden deafness (2

Table III. Abnormal VOR and V-VOR gains in the 86 patients with CNS disorders

Abnormal VOR and V-VOR gains	Cerebellar lesions (n = 23)	Brain stem lesions (n = 34)	Cerebellar and brain stem lesions (n = 29)
VOR ▼ V-VOR ▼	4	*16*	*11*
VOR ▼ or ▲ V-VOR (—)	8	6	4
VOR (—) V-VOR ▼ or ▲	5	4	2
VOR ▲ V-VOR ▲	1	4	2
VOR (—) V-VOR (—)	5	4	10

(—) = Normal;   ▼ = decreased;   ▲ = increased gains

cases), bilateral decreased VOR gains (under 0.37) with slightly decreased OKN and V-VOR were recorded in this test battery. In spite of the frequent presence of spontaneous nystagmus, V-VOR responses were usually symmetric except for only 3 cases with Ménière's disease (2 cases) and sudden deafness (one case at the onset) [8].

FFS Finding in the 133 Patients. There is no observation of FFS finding in caloric nystagmus in the 133 patients with peripheral vestibular disorders.

Patients with CNS Disorders

The OKN, VOR and V-VOR Gains in the 86 Patients with CNS Disorders. Table III shows the division and pathological VOR and V-VOR gains in the 86 patients. According to our normal limits of the OKN, VOR and V-VOR gains (table I), decreased OKN (under 0.73), VOR gains (under 0.57) and V-VOR gains (under 0.80) were frequently observed in patients with combined brain stem cerebellar lesions (10 of 29 cases) and brain stem lesion (16 of 34 cases). On the other hand, bilateral increased VOR gain (over 0.95) with decreased OKN (under 0.73) and normal V-VOR gains (0.80–1.06) was observed in patients with cerebellar lesions (4 of 23 cases).

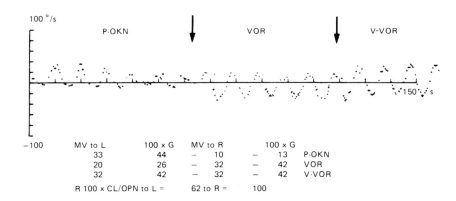

Fig. 1. Pendular rotation in the OK drum in a 64-year-old male.

In some patients with pontine lesions, OKN-DP to the left combined with VOR-DP to the right was recorded, as shown in figure 1. However, low symmetrical V-VOR gains were observed bilaterally. In this case, the visual vestibular modulatory system may not be so much disturbed. This phenomenon suggested that the algebraic summation of the visual and vestibular systems mainly occurred in the cerebellum.

Correlation between the V-VOR Gains and Abnormal FFS of Caloric Nystagmus in the 86 Patients with CNS Disorders. In general, abnormal V-VOR gain was associated with abnormal OKN and FFS finding in caloric nystagmus. However, in some patients with cerebellar and brain stem lesions, we have dissociation findings between the V-VOR and the caloric pattern tests. In the V-VOR test, bilaterally decreased VOR and V-VOR gains (under 0.55) were observed in a patient with cerebellar atrophy. In the caloric pattern test, however, hyperfunction of caloric nystagmus with FFS findings was observed bilaterally.

Therefore, we have analyzed the correlation between the V-VOR gains and the FFS findings of caloric nystagmus. As shown in table IV, in most cases with bilaterally decreased VOR and V-VOR gains, abnormal FFS in caloric nystagmus was more frequently observed. However, in only 3 cases with cerebellar lesions, in one case with brain stem lesions, and in 3 cases with cerebellar and brain stem lesions, FFS with normal V-VOR gain was observed. Therefore, in the cases with cerebellar and brain stem lesions, the

Table IV. Correlation between the VOR and V-VOR gains and abnormal FFS of caloric nystagmus in 86 patients with CNS disorders

FFS positive rate	Cerebellar lesions	Brain stem lesions	Cerebellar and brain stem lesions	Total (26/86)
	6/23 (26%)	9/34 (26%)	11/29 (38%)	
Abnormal V-VOR and VOR	2/5	7/20	7/13	(16/38)
Abnormal V-VOR with normal VOR	1/5	1/4	1/2	(3/11)
Normal V-VOR with abnormal VOR	2/8	0/6	0/4	(2/18)
Normal V-VOR and VOR	1/5	1/4	3/10	(5/19)

V-VOR test could not replace the FFS caloric pattern test, as there is an additional different clinical significance to assess for the modulation of VOR.

Both the OKN, V-VOR test battery and the fixation suppression caloric pattern test are similar evaluation tests for visual vestibular modulation. However, there are some physiological differences between the two test significances from the standpoint of visual vestibular interaction. The V-VOR gain represents the algebraical synergistic summation of the visual and vestibular system. On the other hand, the fixation suppression effect represents the maintaining of gaze stability during vestibular ocular reflex arc.

Moreover, according to Takemori and Cohen [10] and Kato et al. [5] ablation studies in monkeys revealed that total destruction of the flocculus and the nucleus reticularis tegmentis pontis resulted in loss of visual suppression in caloric nystagmus. Therefore, it is generally accepted that the site of visual modulation on vestibular responses is situated in the brain stem and the cerebellum, probably in the vestibulo-cerebellum and its related areas. In the clinical cases, the vestibulo-cerebellum appears to be an important site for visual vestibular modulation that facilitates both short- and long-term adaptive changes in the VOR gain. Furthermore, according to the clinical observations of Kato et al. [6], ENG findings specific to cerebellar lesions were frequently observed as follows: smooth pursuit deficits, dysmetria in saccade accuracy, decreased OKN gain, decreased FS effect in caloric nystagmus, deficits in holding eccentric position, rebound nystagmus and so on. However, ENG finding could not detect any patients who showed neither cerebellar signs nor symptoms.

From our V-VOR gain observation and FFS findings in the patients with vertigo, we have concluded that although the OKN, VOR, V-VOR test battery cannot replace the caloric pattern test, it can provide additional information for evaluation of the visual modulation on VOR. Therefore, we have routinely tested using a combination of the OKN, VOR, V-VOR test battery and the caloric pattern test for evaluation of visual vestibular interaction. However, further studies on the visual vestibular interaction in clinical and experimental cases are needed to identify the localization and laterality of focused lesions.

References

1   Baloh, R.W. et al.: Quantitative assessment of visual-vestibular interaction using sinusoidal rotatory stimuli; in Honrubia, Brazier, Nystagmus and vertigo. Clinical approaches to the patient with dizziness, pp. 231–240 (Academic Press, New York 1982).
2   Honrubia, V. et al.: Identification of the location of vestibular lesions on the basis of vestibulo-ocular reflex measurements. Am. J. Otolaryngol. *1:* 291–301 (1980).
3   Kato, I. et al.: Caloric pattern test with special reference to failure of fixation-suppression. Acta oto-lar. *88:* 97–104 (1979).
4   Kato, I. et al.: Visual-vestibular interaction in central nervous system disorders. Ann. N.Y. Acad. Sci. *374:* 764–773 (1981).
5   Kato, I.; Harada, K.; Nakamura, T.; Sato, Y.; Kawasaki, T.: Role of the nucleus reticularis tegmenti pontis on visually induced eye movements. Expl Neurol. *781:* 503–516 (1982).
6   Kato, I. et al.: Electronystagmographic assessment of cerebellar lesions. Auris Nasus Larynx, Tokyo *13:* suppl. 2, pp. 171–180 (1986).
7   Mizukoshi, K. et al.: Quantitative analysis of the human vestibulo-ocular reflex in sinusoidal rotation. Acta oto-lar., suppl. 393, pp. 58–64 (1983).
8   Mizukoshi, K.; Kobayashi, H.; Ohashi, N.; Watanabe, Y.: Quantitative analysis of the visual vestibulo-ocular reflex using sinusoidal rotation in patients with peripheral vestibular disorders. Acta oto-lar., suppl. 406, pp. 178–181 (1984).
9   Mizukoshi, K. et al.: Quantitative assessment of visual vestibular interaction using sinusoidal rotation in patients with well-defined CNS lesions; in Graham, Kemink, The vestibular system, neuro-physiology and clinical research, pp. 545–554 (Raven Press, New York 1987).
10 Takemori, S.; Cohen, B.: Loss of visual suppression of vestibular nystagmus after flocculus lesions. Brain Res. *72:* 213–224 (1974).

11 Watanabe, Y.; Ohashi, N.; Kobayashi, H.; Takeda, S.; Mizukoshi, K.: Computer analysis of electronystagmography recording in routine equilibrium examinations. Adv. Oto-Rhino-Laryng., vol. 30, pp. 187–192 (Karger, Basel 1983).
12 Wolfe, J.W.; Engelken, E.J.; Olson, J.E.: Low-frequency harmonic acceleration in the evaluation of patients with peripheral labyrinthine disorders; in Honrubia, Brazier, Nystagmus and vertigo, pp. 95–105 (Academic Press, New York 1982).

K. Mizukoshi, MD, Department of Otolaryngology,
Faculty of Medicine, Toyama Medical and Pharmaceutical University,
2630 Sugitani, Toyama City 930-01 (Japan)

Adv. Oto-Rhino-Laryng., vol. 41, pp. 71–75 (Karger, Basel 1988)

Vestibular-Contingent Voluntary Saccades Based on Cognitive Estimates of Remembered Vestibular Information

J. Bloomberg, G. Melvill Jones, B. Segal, S. McFarlane, J. Soul

Aerospace Medical Research Unit, Department of Physiology,
McGill University, Montréal, Qué., Canada

Introduction

Saccades are rapid eye movements that shift gaze (foveal line of regard) to selected targets in space. To achieve this task retinocentric models of saccade generation require only a retinal error signal (target relative to the fovea) to specify saccade direction and amplitude [Schiller and Koerner, 1971]. In addition to a retinal error signal, experiments with head stationary have shown that the saccadic system has access to an internal eye position signal [Hallett and Lightstone, 1976; Sparks and Mays, 1983]. However, in studies of eye-head coordination, where the head is free to move, an additional signal that specifies head movement relative to space is required for saccadic gaze control [Guitton et al., 1984; Guitton and Volle 1987; Laurutis and Robinson, 1986].

The aim of the present study was to determine if saccades could be made, in the dark, to a just-viewed target based on remembered *vestibular* information. The existence of this capability would suggest a functionally meaningful vestibular access to the saccade generating mechanism.

Methods

Nine subjects aged 18–63 participated in these experiments. Subjects sat on a servo-controlled rotating chair with head fixed to it by a dental bite. First (fig. 1), a central earth-

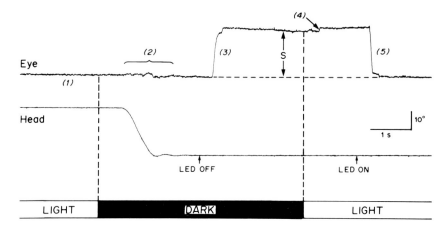

Fig. 1. Vestibular-contingent saccade test. (1) Subject visually fixates the earth-fixed target. (2) Fixation is then transferred to the head-fixed LED to suppress the VOR during chair rotation in the dark. (3) Following chair rotation the LED is turned off signaling the subject to make a saccade, in darkness, to the perceived location of the earth-fixed target. (4) In the light, a corrective saccade is made, if required, onto the earth-fixed target. (5) The head-fixed LED is re-fixated. S represents the cumulated amplitude of the vestibular-contingent saccade(s).

fixed target was visually fixated. Fixation was then transferred to a head-fixed low intensity LED target just under the first. The lights were then extinguished and the subject was passively rotated to the right or left at 40 °/s through one of six randomly chosen angular amplitudes (5–30°) while suppressing the vestibulo-ocular reflex (VOR) by fixating on the head-fixed target. After cessation of head rotation, the head-fixed LED was extinguished signaling the subject to voluntarily fixate, in total darkness, the internally perceived location of the earth-fixed target. Finally, in the light, the actual earth-fixed target was re-foveated to record the oculomotor error and to establish the electro-oculographic calibration for each individual test. Each test was repeated 5 times for each amplitude and direction for a total of 60 tests per subject. Eye movements were minimized by fixation on the head-fixed LED to control for change in eye position with respect to the head during rotation.

A potential problem arises from the fact that head movement during visual suppression of eye movement can induce adaptive reduction in the gain of the VOR [Miles and Eighmy, 1980]. To monitor this potentially confounding effect, slow phase VOR gain was measured before and after the testing series, using methods previously described by Segal and Katsarkas [1988]. In addition, the effects of *post*-test visual positional feedback of actual oculomotor error was examined by repeating a complete series of vestibular-contingent saccade tests without such feedback in 4 of the original 9 subjects (i.e. excluding step 4 in fig. 1).

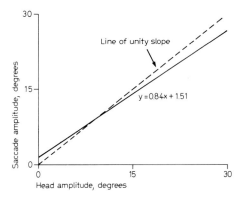

Fig. 2. Relationship between cumulative vestibular-contingent saccade amplitude and amplitude of preceding change in head rotational position for all subjects combined. Continuous line: regression line fitted to all the data; dashed line: line through unity slope and zero intercept.

Chair position, and hence position of the head was obtained from a precision (1% full scale error) potentiometer located in the axis of chair rotation. Horizontal eye position was recorded by means of DC coupled electro-oculography. Both eye and chair signals were low pass filtered at 100 Hz and computer sampled at 300 Hz (D.E.C. 11/23).

Results

Figure 1 shows the performance of one subject during a single vestibular-contingent saccade test. The cumulative amplitude (S in fig. 1) of vestibular-contingent saccades, made in total darkness, was 93% of ideal; thus, only a small corrective visual saccade was required to re-foveate the actual earth-fixed target in the light.

Figure 2 shows cumulative saccade amplitude versus the change in preceding head rotational position (head amplitude) for all subjects and tests combined. A straight line fitted to all the data (continuous line in fig. 2) had a slope of 0.84 ± 0.04 (mean ± standard error of mean) and a y intercept of 1.51 ± 0.39. Saccade amplitude was significantly ($p < 0.001$) positively correlated ($r = 0.91$; $n = 533$) with amplitude of head movement. The slope of 0.84 indicates that the cumulative saccade size was consistently close to, but slightly less than ideal. This deviation from unity was the result of small saccades (5°) tending to be slightly greater than ideal (i.e. overshooting the target) and large saccades (30°) tending to be slightly less than ideal (i.e. undershooting the target).

There was no significant difference in mean slow phase VOR gain estimated before (0.79 ± 0.02) and after (0.78 ± 0.02) the vestibular-contingent saccade testing. There was also no significant difference in tests performed with and without post-test visual feedback of oculomotor error in the 4 subjects exposed to these two conditions.

Discussion

The results demonstrate that subjects can generate appropriate volitional ocular saccades, in the dark, to a just-viewed target following a step change of head rotational position conducted in the dark. Since the saccades were generated in total darkness and eye movements during rotation were suppressed, it is inferred that the memory of the vestibular response to head rotation provided the necessary input to the saccadic system to specify the appropriate saccadic parameters. Hence, it is inferred that memorized vestibular information can access the saccade generating system.

Vestibular input integrated with respect to time could provide a signal specifying head movement relative to space. This signal combined with retinotopic and craniotopic (eye re head) signals could provide the necessary information for generating goal-directed saccadic shifts in gaze relative to inertial space in the presence of head movement.

The saccadic system may be subject to adaptive change when confronted with altered visual feedback [Optican, 1985]. However, the vestibular-contingent saccades of our experiment, were unaffected by the presence of post-test visual feedback of oculomotor error, at least in the 4 subjects examined for this purpose. Thus, a memory of post-test *visual* feedback was not apparently used to improve saccadic performance. Also, there was no detectable change of slow phase VOR gain over the course of these experiments, presumably due to the very short durations of visual VOR suppression (0.1–0.6 s per test).

Subjects made volitional saccades to the internally perceived location of the earth-fixed target after completion of a step change in head rotational position in the dark. The saccade performance was therefore based upon a cognitive perception of the vestibular response to head rotation. Thus, these vestibular-contingent saccades presumably represent the volitional response to a perceptual correlate of vestibular function.

References

Guitton, D.; Douglas, R.M.; Volle, M.: Eye-head coordination in the cat. J. Neurophysiol. *52:* 1030–1050 (1984).

Guitton, D.; Volle, M.: Gaze control in humans: eye-head coordination during orienting movements to targets within and beyond the oculomotor range. J. Neurophysiol. *58:* 427–459 (1987).

Hallett, P.E.; Lightstone, A.D.: Saccadic eye movements toward stimuli triggered by prior saccades. Vision Res. *16:* 99–106 (1976).

Laurutis, V.P.; Robinson, D.A.: The vestibulo-ocular reflex during saccadic eye movement. J. Physiol. *373:* 209–233 (1986).

Miles, F.A.; Eighmy, B.B.: Long-term adaptive changes in primate vestibulo-ocular reflex. I. Behavioural observations. J. Neurophysiol. *43:* 1406–1425 (1980).

Optican, L.M.: Adaptive properties of the saccadic system; in Berthoz, Melvill Jones, Adaptive mechanisms in gaze control, pp. 71–78 (Elsevier/Biomedical Press, Amsterdam 1985).

Segal, B.H.; Katsarkas, A.: Goal directed vestibulo-ocular function in man: gaze stabilization by slow-phase and saccadic eye movements. Exp. Brain Res. *70:* 26–32 (1988).

Schiller, P.H.; Koerner, F.: Discharge characteristics of single units in superior colliculus of the alert rhesus monkey. J. Neurophysiol. *34:* 920–936 (1971).

Sparks, D.L.; Mays, L.E.: Spatial localization of saccade targets. I. Compensation of stimulation-induced perturbations in eye position. J. Neurophysiol. *49:* 45–63 (1983).

J. Bloomberg, Aerospace Medical Research Unit, Department of Physiology, McGill University, Montréal, Qué. H3G 1Y6 (Canada)

Adv. Oto-Rhino-Laryng., vol. 41, pp. 76–81 (Karger, Basel 1988)

Linear Displacement Can Be Derived from Otolithic Information and Stored on Spatial Maps Controlling the Saccadic System

Alain Berthoz[a], Isabelle Israël[a]. Elisabeth Vitte[b], David Zee[c]

[a]Laboratoire de Physiologie Neurosensorielle, CNRS, Paris, France;
[b]Hôpital Lariboisière (Service Prof. Freyss), Paris, France;
[c]Johns Hopkins Hospital, Baltimore, Md., USA

Introduction

It is well known that the otolith-ocular reflex induced by linear acceleration has an extremely weak gain [2, 3, 7, 10]. However, the otoliths seem to be able to modulate the gain of oculomotor reflexes induced by head rotation [5], optokinetic stimulation [2, 8], visual target pursuit [3], or acoustic target tracking [3]. Even though the otolith-ocular gain is small, it seems that the information provided by the otoliths is indeed taken into account during multisensorial stimulation, and is processed and integrated into other oculomotor control subsystems.

The aim of the present experiment was to assess the ability of the CNS to derive linear displacement from a 'pure' otolithic stimulation. We observed the tracking eye movements of the mental image of an earth-fixed target executed by subjects submitted to a horizontal linear acceleration.

Preliminary account of the response to sinusoidal stimulation has been published elsewhere [1].

Methods

Subjects were seated in a motorised cart (linear acceleration device), which induced head movements along the y-axis. The head was held by a helmet fixed to the chair inside the cart, and kept in complete darkness during the experiments. An earth-fixed target was adjusted at eye level for each subject. Distance from the subject to the target on the x-axis

was constant (63 cm). Maximum cart displacement amplitude used here was about
100 cm, and maximum acceleration about 1 m/s (0.15 g). Only horizontal eye movements were measured with DC EOG (cut-off frequency: 200 Hz).

Four healthy subjects and 4 bilabyrinthectomized patients (bilateral acoustic neuromas) participated in the experiments. The healthy subjects wore headphones generating a
white noise so that no auditory cues were available to them. Three different sets of tests
were executed by each subject.

Sine Wave Test. The velocity command sent to the cart was a sine wave (SW) of
0.22 Hz frequency and unpredictable amplitude. At least 6 different amplitudes of stimulation were randomly applied. The subject had first to identify the fixed target in front of
him. Then the light was turned off and the cart set in motion. The subject had been
instructed to remember and/or imagine the earth-fixed target initially placed in front of
him and to keep his eyes on it, i.e. to track the mental image of the target during his own
displacement. After about 5 cycles of SW stimulation, light went on and the subject had to
track the now visible target (smooth pursuit) during some more cycles, providing direct
calibration of the EOG recordings.

On-Line Step Test. A 0.2-Hz SW velocity command was used. The stimulation
stopped after one half-cycle, leading to a damped step of head position. As in the SW
experiment, the subject was shown the earth-fixed target, then light was turned off, and the
cart set in motion. The subject had to track the mental image of the target during the cart
displacement. About 1 s after the cart had stopped, light went on and the cart was driven
back to its initial position. The subject smoothly tracked the now visible target, again
providing calibration of the EOG signals.

Memorized Steps Test. Stimulation was the same as for the on-line step (OLS) test.
The subject first identified the fixed target in front of him. When the light was turned off,
he was instructed to keep his eyes in the primary position, i.e. to keep his gaze right in
front of him during the displacement. After the cart had stopped and after a variable delay
of 5–50 s, the subject was asked to saccade back to the earth-fixed target, still in darkness.
Then light went on, and the subject made, if needed, a corrective saccade to the now
visible target. The cart was driven back to the initial position while the subject smoothly
tracked the target to the end. This test was only performed by healthy subjects.

Results

Sine Wave Test

Healthy Subjects. Eye tracking movements consisted in saccades, separated by short slow phases (fig. 1). Only one subject could smoothly track the
imagined target, during short periods of time. Cumulative slow phase
position was plotted and found to be directed opposite to subject motion and
reversed periodically with the same frequency as subject oscillations. Its

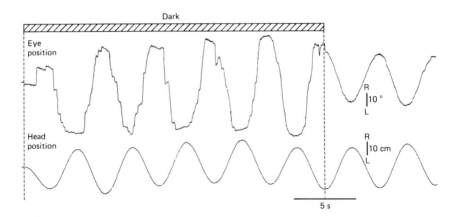

Fig. 1. Recording of horizontal eye movements during sinusoidal linear acceleration (SW test). Top trace: angular eye position (degrees). Bottom trace: linear position of the moving cart (cm). Before cart motion the subject is in light and sees the target at 63 cm distance in front of him. During cart motion in the dark, he tries to keep gaze on the imagined/memorized earth-fixed target. When the light is turned on again, the subject pursues the now visible earth-fixed target.

peak-to-peak amplitude never exceeded 12° (corresponding to a mean VOR gain of about 0.12 °/cm). Phase ranged between 190 and 260° with respect to head position.

Amplitude of cart displacement was fairly well reproduced by all subjects. Quantitative results concerning this condition have been published elsewhere [1]. All subjects more or less overestimated the displacement amplitude (fig. 1). Overestimation was maximal for lower stimulations (up to 350%).

Bilabyrinthectomized Patients. In order to exclude the contribution of somatosensory cues to the observed eye movements, the same experiment was performed with 4 patients suffering from bilateral acoustic neuromas. A typical example of record obtained on one of these patients in shown on figure 2a. During cart motion in darkness, the subject is obviously unable to track the target. It is particularly interesting that even in these patients, who are probably accustomed to use somatosensory cues as a substitute for the defective labyrinths, the response is absent. Figure 2b shows a quantitative measurement of the peak-to-peak eye movements versus head peak-to-peak displacement amplitude for the 4 patients.

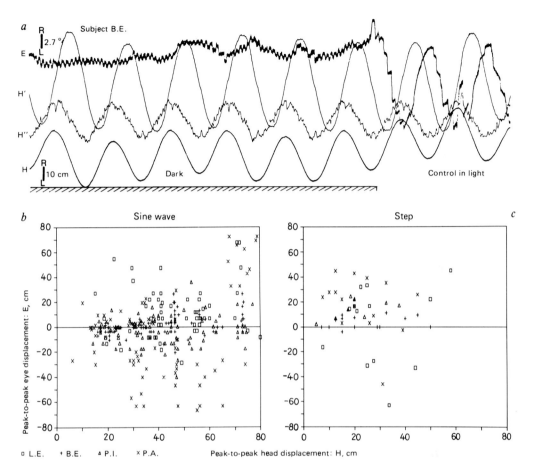

Fig. 2. Tracking of an earth-fixed target by bilabyrinthectomized patients. *a* Recordings of eye position E (degrees), head position H (cm), velocity H' (cm/s) and acceleration H" (cm/s^2) during sinusoidal linear motion. *b* Relationship between peak-to-peak eye displacement and peak-to-peak head displacement during sinusoidal linear cart motion at 0.22 Hz (SW test). *c* Same as in *b*, during steps (OLS) test.

On-Line Steps Test

Healthy Subjects. As in the SW test, subjects tracked the target with saccades. Their assessment of the cart direction and amplitude was still better than during the SW test.

Bilabyrinthectomized Patients. Patients were not able to assess the cart displacement amplitude during this test either. Some of them tried to guess the ongoing displacement amplitude and direction using the information provided by the control (cart driven back in light) of the preceding step. Figure 2c shows the quantitative measurements of the eye movements during cart motion. This plot illustrates the lack of estimation of the displacement by these patients.

Memorized Steps Test (Healthy Subjects Only)

The performance of the subjects in reproducing cart displacement was almost as good as during OLS test. There was no effect of the time interval (5–50 s) between the end of cart displacement and the instruction to gaze at the presumed position of the target in this performance.

Conclusion

These results provide the first demonstration of the fact that otolith-derived information concerning head linear displacement can be stored and retrieved by the brain. The fact that bilabyrinthectomized patients do not show this property establishes the true vestibular origin of this ability. We have to assume that a double integration of the linear acceleration detected by the otoliths is performed, or that velocity storage can be used to induce a position command. These results are very much in accordance with those obtained by Melvill Jones et al. [9; and this volume] on angular acceleration. They provide a new way to test the otolithic function.

References

1   Berthoz, A.; Israel, I.; Viéville, T.; Zee, D.: Linear head displacement measured by the otoliths can be reproduced through the saccadic system. Neurosci. Lett. *82:* 285–290 (1987).
2   Buizza, A.; Léger, A.; Droulez, J.; Berthoz, A.; Schmid, R.: Influence of otolithic stimulation by horizontal linear acceleration on optokinetic nystagmus and visual motion perception. Exp. Brain Res. *39:* 165–176 (1980).
3   Buizza, A.; Schmid, R.; Droulez, J.: Influence of linear acceleration on oculomotor control; in Fuchs, Becker, Progress in oculomotor research, pp. 524–527 (Elsevier, New York 1981).
4   Chun, K.S.; Robinson, D.A.: A model of quick phase generation in the vestibulo-ocular reflex. Biol. Cybernet. *28:* 209–221 (1978).

5   Gresty, M.; Bronstein, A.M.; Barratt, H.: Eye movement responses to combined linear and angular head movement. Exp. Brain Res. *65:* 377–384 (1987).
6   Guedry, R.E.; Harris, C.S.: Labyrinthine function related to experiments on the parallel swing. NASA Joint Report — Order No. R-93, Bureau of Medicine and Surgery — Project MR005.13-6001, 1963.
7   Lichtenberg, B.K.; Young, L.R.; Arrott, A.P.: Human ocular counterrolling induced by varying linear accelerations. Exp. Brain Res. *48:* 127–136 (1982).
8   Matsuo, V.; Cohen, B.: Vertical optokinetic nystagmus and vestibular nystagmus in the monkey. Up-down asymmetry and effects of gravity. Exp. Brain Res. *53:* 197–216 (1984).
9   Melvill Jones, G.; Bloomberg, J.; Segal, B.; McFarlane, S.; Soul, J.: Vestibular-contingent ocular saccades to remembered visual targets. Abstract of Canadian Physiological Society, June 1987, Ste Adele, Quebec.
10   Niven, S.I.; Hixson, C.E.; Correia, M.J.: Elicitation of horizontal nystagmus by periodical acceleration. Acta oto-lar. *62:* 429–441 (1985).

Alain Berthoz, Laboratoire de Physiologie Neurosensorielle,
CNRS, F–75270 Paris Cedex 06 (France)

Adv. Oto-Rhino-Laryng., vol. 41, pp. 82–88 (Karger, Basel 1988)

Compensatory Eye Movement Gain and Head-Eye Latencies Change with Verbal Feedback: Voluntary Adjustment of Gaze Types

W.H. Zangemeister, D. Schlüter, K. Kunze

Neurological University Clinic Hamburg, Hamburg, FRG

Introduction

For some time it has been known that visual and mental effort influence the vestibular ocular reflex (VOR). Besides visual long- and short-term adaptation to reversing prisms [Melvill Jones and Gonshor, 1982] and fixation suppression of the VOR [Takemori and Cohen, 1974; Dichgans et al., 1978; Zangemeister and Hansen 1986], the mental set of a subject can influence the VOR, e.g. through an imagined target [Barr et al., 1976; Melvill Jones et al., 1984] or anticipatory intent only [Zangemeister and Stark, 1981]. In contrast to animals, human head and eye movements are governed by a conscious will of the human performer, that includes verbal communication. Thus, in a given experimental setup the synkinesis of active human gaze may be changed according to instruction. The verbal feedback to the subject might permit to generate the whole range of gaze types, even with amplitude and prediction of a visual target being constant.

The gaze types [Zangemeister and Stark, 1982a] are defined by head minus eye latency differences (see Methods). This has been demonstrated particularly by looking at the timing of the neck electromyogram as the head movement control signal [Zangemeister et al., 1982; Zangemeister and Stark, 1983; Stark et al., 1986].

In this study, we compared the voluntarily changeable human gaze types performed during the same experiment without and with the addition of a randomly applied perturbation to the head-eye movement system. We tried to answer three questions in particular: (1) Are we able to modulate continuously the types of coordinated gaze through conscious intent during predictive active head movements? (2) How is the gaze (saccade and VOR/

CEM [compensatory eye movement] response to passive random head rotation from zero head velocity with respect to the preset intent of a given subject? (3) Does random perturbation of the head during the early phase of gaze acceleration generate responses that are the sum of responses to experiment (1) and (2)?

Methods

Eye movements were recorded by monocular DC electro-oculography, head movements by using a horizontal angular accelerometer (Schaevitz) and a high resolution ceramic potentiometer linked to the head through universal joints [Zangemeister and Stark, 1982b]. Twelve normal subjects (age 22–25) attended a semicircular screen sitting in a darkened room. While they actively performed fast horizontal (saccadic) head rotations between two continuously lit targets at ± 30° amplitude with a frequency around 0.3 Hz, they were instructed to focus on the following tasks: (a) 'shift your eyes ahead of your head', (b) 'shift your head ahead of your eyes'. During (a) they were instructed to shift the eyes 'long before' (i, type II), or 'shortly before' (ii, type I) the head. During (b) they were instructed to shift the head 'earlier' (i, type IIIA), or 'much earlier' (ii, type IIIB) than the eyes, eventually 'with the intent to suppress any eye movement' (type IIIB or IV). Each task included 50–100 head movements. Gaze types were defined by eye minus head latency (ms). Type: II < 50; I = 50; IIIa > 50–200; IIIb > 200–550; IV > 550. Perturbations were done pseudorandomly: (a) from a zero P, V, A (position, velocity, acceleration) initial condition of the head-eye movement system, (b) during the early phase of head acceleration. They consisted of (a) fast passive head accelerations, (b) of short decelerating or accelerating impulses during the early phase of active head acceleration and were recorded by the head-mounted accelerometer. Perturbation impulses were generated through an apparatus that permitted manual acceleration or deceleration of the head through cords that were tangentially linked directly to the tightly set head helmet.

Results

Subjects demonstrated their ability (fig. 1a) to switch between gaze types in the experimentally set predictive situation of constant and large amplitude targets. The respective gains (eye/head velocity) were: type II 0.9–1.1, type III 0.13, type IV 0.06–0.09. This result was expected from earlier studies [Zangemeister and Huefner, 1984; Zangemeister and Stark, 1982a, b]. Our subjects showed differing amounts of success in performing the intended gaze type, with type IV being the most difficult to perform, supposedly because of its highest concentration necessary: type II 76%; type I 56%; type III 69%; type IV 16%.

Random perturbation of the head while in primary position with head velocity and acceleration being zero (fig. 2) resulted in large saccades/quick

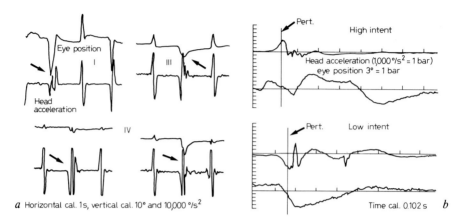

a Horizontal cal. 1 s, vertical cal. 10° and 10,000 °/s²   *b*

Fig. 1. a Gaze types I, II, IV generated intentionally through verbal feedback (without arrows); random perturbation of gaze type I, III, IV in flight (arrows). *b* Random perturbation of gaze type III with high (upper) and low (lower) intent; compare figure 3 for gaze pursuit and intent.

phases of long duration, and a large and delayed VOR/CEM, if the subject had low preset intent to withstand the perturbation; in this case head acceleration showed a long-lasting damped oscillation. With increasing intent of the subject head acceleration became finally highly overdamped, but still with comparable initial acceleration values, and eye movements showed increasingly smaller and shorter quick phases as well as an early short VOR response. In addition, with the highest intent a late anticompensatory eye movement was obtained.

Random perturbations of the accelerating head, i.e. sudden acceleration or deceleration of gaze in flight (fig. 1a, b arrows), were characterized by small VOR responses after the perturbation in the case of high intent of the subject as in gaze type IIIB, or much higher VOR/CEM gain in the case of low intent comparable to gaze type I. Respective gains were (fig. 1a): type I 0.55, type III 0.06, type IV 0.08 (left), 0.09 (right); (fig. 1b): 0.13 (upper), 0.90 (lower).

Random perturbations were also applied during coordinated head-eye pursuit movements of a sinusoidally moving target (maximum velocity 50 deg/s.) with the VOR being suppressed through constant fixation of the pursuit target. Figure 3 demonstrates the different amount of VOR fixation suppression as a function of changing intent during fixation of a sinusoidal target of the same frequency.

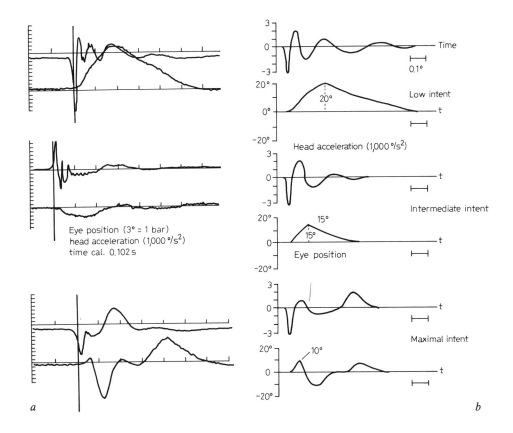

Fig. 2. a Random perturbation from primary position, low (uppermost), interme-diate (middle), high (lowermost) intent. *b* Random perturbation from primary position, explanatory scheme.

Discussion

The three initial questions could be answered as follows: In non-random situations subjects can intentionally and continuously change their gaze types. Gaze responses to passive random head accelerations depend on the subject's preset intent. Perturbation of predictive gaze saccades in midflight results in the sum of task one and two.

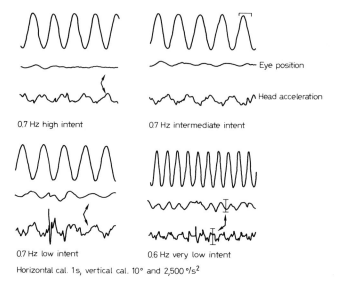

Horizontal cal. 1s, vertical cal. 10° and 2,500 °/s^2

Fig. 3. Variable amount of fixation suppression of the VOR as a function of intent during gaze pursuit of the same target frequency.

The input-output characteristics of the VOR are subject to major moment-to-moment fluctuations depending on non-visual factors, such as state of 'arousal' [Melvill Jones and Sugie, 1972] and mental set [Collins, 1962]. More recently, it has been found that the influence of 'mental set' depends explicitly upon the subject's conscious choice of intended visual goal [Barr et al., 1976; Sharpe et al., 1981; Baloh et al., 1984; Fuller et al., 1983], i.e. following earth-fixed or head-fixed targets during head rotation. Consistent alteration of the mentally chosen goal can alone produce adaptive alteration of internal parameters controlling VOR gain [Berthoz and Melvill Jones, 1985]. Obviously, comparison of afferent retinal slip detectors with concurrent vestibular afferents can be substituted by a 'working' comparison made between the vestibular input and an efferent feedback copy of either the concurrent or the imagined or anticipated concurrent oculomotor output, as proposed by Miles and Lisberger [1981].

Our results presented here demonstrate the ability of the subjects to perform short-term adaptation during verbal feedback instructing for eye-head latency changes that changed the types of active gaze. These results are comparable to the data from Barr et al. [1976], in that an almost immediate change between different VOR gains with constant visual input could be generated. In addition, our perturbation experiments expanded these data demonstrating the task- (or gaze-type) dependent attenuation of the VOR. This is in contrast to results in animals, where perturbation of visually triggered eye-head saccades resulted in an acceleration of the eye [Guitton et al., 1984; Fuller et al., 1983], because a conscious task-influence of the VOR is impossible. Therefore, not only a representation of the target's percept [Barr et al., 1976] can be created, but also an internal image of the anticipated VOR response in conjunction with the appropriate saccade.

We hypothesize that through the cortico-cerebellar loop a given subject is able to continuously eliminate the VOR response during predictive gaze movements. This is done internally be generating an image of the anticipated VOR response in conjunction with the appropriate saccade, and then subtracting it from the actual reflex response. This internal image can be manipulated intentionally and continuously *without* a VOR on/off switch. In this way a flexible adaptation of the conscious subject to anticipated tasks is performed.

References

Barr, C.C.; Schultheis, L.; Robinson, D.A.: Voluntary, non-visual control of the human vestibulo-ocular reflex. Acta oto-lar. *81:* 365–375 (1976).

Collins, W.E.: Effects of mental set upon vestibular nystagmus. J. exp. Psychol. *63:* 191-197 (1962).

Dichgans, J.; Reutern, G.v.; Römmelt, U.: Impaired suppression of vestibular nystagmus by fixation. Arch. Psychiat. Nerv. Krankh. *226:* 183-199 (1978).

Fuller, J.H.; Maldonado, H.; Schlag, J.: Vestibular-oculomotor interaction in cat eye-head movements. Exp. Brain Res. *271:* 241–250 (1983).

Guitton, D.; Douglas, R.; Valle, M.: Eye-head coordination in cats. J. Neurophysiol. *52:* 1030–1050 (184).

Melvill Jones, G.; Berthoz, A.; Segal, B.: Adaptive modification of the vestibulo-ocular reflex by mental effort in darkness. Exp. Brain Res. *56:* 149–153 (1984).

Melvill Jones, G.; Gonshor, A.: Oculomotor response to rapid head oscillation after prolonged adaptation to vision reversal. Exp. Brain Res. *45:* 45–58 (1982).

Stark, L.; Zangemeister, W.H.; Hannaford, B.; Kunze, K.: Use of models of brainstem reflexes for clinical research; in Kunze, Zangemeister, Arlt, Clinical problems of brainstem disorders, pp. 172–184 (Thieme, Stuttgart 1986).

Takemori, S.; Cohen, B.: Loss of visual suppression of vestibular nystagmus after flocculus lesions. Brain Res. *72:* 213–224 (1974).

Zangemeister, W.H.; Hansen, H.C.: Fixation suppression of the vestibular ocular reflex and head movement correlated EEG potentials; in O'Reagan, Levy-Schoen, Eye movements, pp. 247–256 (Elsevier, Amsterdam 1986).

Zangemeister, W.H.; Huefner, G.: Saccades during active head movements: interactive gaze types; in Gale, Johnson, Theoretical and applied aspects of eye movement research, pp. 113–122 (Elsevier, Amsterdam 1984).

Zangemeister, W.H.; Stark, L.: Active head rotation and eye-head coordination; in Cohen, Vestibular and oculomotor physiology. Ann. N.Y. Acad. Sci. *374:* 540-559 (1981).

Zangemeister, W.H.; Stark, L.: Gaze types: interactions of eye and head movements in gaze. Expl Neurol. *77:* 563–577 (1982a).

Zangemeister, W.H.; Stark, L.: Gaze latency: variable interactions of eye and head in gaze. Expl Neurol. *75:* 389–406 (1982b).

Zangemeister, W.H.; Stark, L.: Pathological types of eye and head gaze coordination. Neuro-ophthalmol. *3:* 259-276 (1983).

Zangemeister, W.H.; Stark, .; Meienberg, O.; Waite, T.: Motor control of head movements. J. neurol. Sci. *55:* 1–14 (1982).

Prof. Dr. med. W.H. Zangemeister, Neurological University Clinic Hamburg, Martinistrasse 52, D–2000 Hamburg 20 (FRG)

Adv. Oto-Rhino-Laryng., vol. 41, pp. 89–94 (Karger, Basel 1988)

The Role of the Vestibular System in Eye-Head Coordination and the Generation of Vestibular Nystagmus[1]

R. Schmid, D. Zambarbieri

Dipartimento di Informatica e Sistemistica, Università di Pavia, Pavia, Italy

Introduction

The vestibulo-ocular reflex (VOR) has been developed to make the eyes a stable platform for vision. When head rotations are produced in total darkness, there is no need of compensatory eye movement. Nevertheless, they take place. Why, in this condition, is VOR not inhibited?

The results of the many studies on VOR adaptation to modified visual or environmental conditions [Berthoz and Melvill Jones, 1985] and those on VOR gain control during eye-head orientation [Laurutis and Robinson, 1986; Pelisson and Prablanc, 1986] have shown that the central nervous system (CNS) can produce not only long-term modifications of VOR but also on-line inhibition. Why is this inhibition not produced during vestibular stimulation in darkness? Which is the current CNS strategy underlying the eye movement control that leads in darkness to a nystagmic response?

Good suggestions are not missing in the literature [Melvill Jones, 1964; Mishkin and Melvill Jones, 1966; Barnes and Benson, 1973; Schmid and Lardini, 1976; Chun and Robinson, 1978], but so far they received little attention. On the other hand, only the recent studies on the role of the vestibular system in gaze control during eye-head movements seem to provide the experimental evidence for a correct interpretation of vestibular nystagmus.

[1] Work supported by MPI and CNR, Nucleo per le Applicazioni Biomediche dei Calcolatori.

The aim of this paper is to review the main relevant results of these studies and to show how they can be used to construct a model of eye movement control that justifies the occurrence of nystagmus during a vestibular stimulation in darkness.

The Role of the Vestibular System in Eye-Head Coordination

When a subject is presented with a visual target in a free head condition and target eccentricity does not exceed 30°, gaze fixation is accomplished through a coordinated eye-head movement in which the eyes make a saccade to the target a few milliseconds before the beginning of head movement. Gaze stability is then maintained by a slow eye movement that compensates the head movement [Morasso et al., 1973]. The role of the vestibular system in this condition is to provide the VOR with the input necessary for compensation.

An additional role was revealed when the experiments were performed with more eccentric targets or when orienting head movements were produced in the dark. In these cases the eyes made a saccade after the beginning of head movement. It was therefore suggested that the output of the vestibular system can also be used to program the eye fixation saccade [Barnes, 1979]. A more conclusive evidence was obtained when the profile of a natural head movement was reproduced in darkness by a passive rotation of the head on the trunk [Barnes, 1979] and by a passive rotation of the body in toto [Roucoux et al., 1981]. In either condition, an input to the saccadic system through an efference copy of the head motor command can be excluded. In the latter case, also an input from neck proprioceptors can be excluded. The reafferent vestibular signal is therefore the only source of information that can be used to command the saccadic eye movement that brings the eyes where the head is moving to, 200–300 ms after the onset of head movement.

The functional significance of such a vestibular input to the saccadic system is quite clear. In natural orientation head movements, the head takes about 500 ms to reach the intended position, a time too long in many instances. It is better to estimate where the head is going and throw the eyes close to this position. Since in natural orientation head movements there is a linear relationship between the amplitude of head rotation and peak head velocity [Zangemeister et al., 1981], an estimate of the former can be obtained from the latter. Peak head velocity is reached after less than 200 ms from the onset of head movement and during this time the frequency discharge of primary vestibular neurons reproduces the profile of head velocity very precisely. Thus, within the first 200 ms the CNS receives from the vestibular system all the information needed to compute an appropriate saccadic eye movement. Darkness would not be a reason enough to exclude this strategy of eye-head coordination. When the head is moved in darkness towards a point of interest, it is not known whether a visible object is actually present in this position or not.

A Model of Eye-Head Coordination in the Dark and the Generation of Vestibular Nystagmus

The results reviewed in the previous section suggest the existence of a vestibulo-saccadic pathway (VSP) which is used in a reflex way during large orientation head movements both in the light and in darkness. To pick up a value of the vestibular output that roughly corresponds to head peak velocity and therefore proportional to the intended head deviation, VSP should be made active after about 200 ms from the onset of head rotation. Moreover, in order to avoid undesired saccades in the direction of head movement when a slow compensatory eye movement is actually needed to maintain the fixation of a stationary target, it is likely that a threshold exists on the value of the vestibular output able to activate VSP. The model shown in figure 1 can then be proposed. The gain of VSP would represent the proportionality factor of about 0.4 °/°/s between amplitude and peak velocity in fast orientation head movements. The saturation of VSP excludes that saccades are commanded beyond the mechanical limits of eye rotation in the orbit. Finally, a threshold control on the input to the saccadic mechanism has been represented to account for the temporary inhibition of this mechanism after each saccade.

When a vestibular stimulation is produced in the dark as in current clinical rotary tests, the following pattern of response can be predicted. The beginning of the response is always a compensatory movement, the minimum duration of which is the delay of the mechanism for VSP activation. Once the VSP has been activated, the output of the vestibular receptors, appropriately scaled and limited, is sent to the saccadic mechanism as *reference signal*. A first saccade is produced in the anticompensatory direction with an amplitude that depends on the value of the vestibular output at the time of VSP activation and on eye position relative to the head at that time. After this first saccade, the saccadic mechanism remains inhibited for a

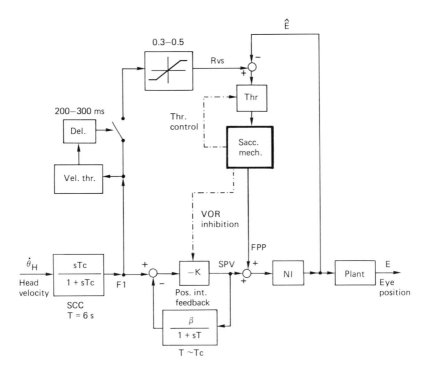

Fig. 1. Model of vestibular nystagmus generation. SCC = Semicircular canals; Rvs = reference signal to the saccadic mechanism; F1 = discharge frequency of primary vestibular neurons; SPV = slow phase velocity; FPP = fast phase pulses; NI = neural integrator.

while and a slow compensatory movement can take place. As soon as the saccadic mechanism is enabled again, a second saccade is produced which brings the eyes to the position indicated by the vestibular input to the saccadic mechanism at that time, and so on. A *nystagmic response* is then predicted. Also the predominance of the anticompensatory phase as described by Melvill Jones [1964] for post-rotational responses and by Mishkin and Melvill Jones [1966] for sinusoidal responses can be predicted accurately.

The important two points with this interpretation of vestibular nystagmus are, first, the active part of the response is actually the fast phase and not the slow phase; second, the eye position at the end of each fast phase should be a discrete time representation of the output of the vestibular system.

Conclusion

The results of the last years' studies on eye-head coordination during fast orienting head movements provide a basis for the interpretation of the nystagmic response evoked by vestibular stimulation in the dark. According to this interpretation, the fast phase of nystagmus would reflect a strategy of eye-head coordination by which the eyes are thrown where the head is moving to in order to pick up quickly an object of interest. Thus, the fast phase of nystagmus has not the simple function of resetting the eyes to the central position, but it is likely to represent the active part of the response. A VSP bringing a signal proportional to the discharge frequency of primary vestibular neurons to the saccadic system should be assumed. The eye position at the end of each fast phase of nystagmus would provide a discrete representation of the VSP signal and therefore a direct estimate of the function of the peripheral vestibular system.

References

Barnes, G.R.: Vestibulo-ocular function during head and eye movements to acquire visual targets. J. Physiol. *287:* 127–147 (1979).

Barnes, G.R.; Benson, A.J.: A model for the prediction of the nystagmic response to angular and linear acceleration stimuli: in NATO AGARD CCP-128. The use of nystagmography in aviation medicine, A23, 1–13 (1973).

Berthoz, A.; Melvill Jones, G.: Adaptive mechanisms in gaze control. Facts and theories. Reviews of oculomotor research, vol. 1 (Elsevier, Amsterdam 1985).

Chun, K.S.; Robinson, D.A.: A model of quick phase generation in the vestibulo-ocular reflex. Biol. Cybern. *28:* 209–221 (1978).

Laurutis, V.P.; Robinson, D.A.: The vestibulo-ocular reflex during human saccadic eye movements. J. Physiol. *373:* 209–233 (1986).

Melvill Jones, G.: Predominance of anticompensatory oculomotor response during rapid head rotation. Aerospace Med. *35:* 965–968 (1964).

Mishkin, S.; Melvill Jones, G.: Predominant direction of gaze during slow head rotation. Aerospace Med. *37:* 897–900 (1966).

Morasso, P.; Bizzi, E.; Dichgans, J.: Adjustment of saccade characteristics during head movements. Exp. Brain Res. *16:* 492–500 (1973).

Pelisson, D.; Prablanc, C.: Vestibulo-ocular reflex (VOR) induced by passive head rotation and goal directed saccadic eye movements do not simply add in man. Brain Res. *380:* 397–400 (1986).

Roucoux, A.; Crommelinck, M.; Guerit, J.M.; Meulders, M.: Two modes of eye-head coordination and the role of the vestibulo-ocular reflex in these two strategies; in Fuchs, Becker, Progress in oculomotor research, pp. 309–315 (Elsevier/North-Holland, Amsterdam 1981).

Schmid, R.; Lardini, F.: On the predominance of anti-compensatory eye movements in vestibular nystagmus. Biol. Cybern. *23:* 135–148 (1976).

Zangemeister, W.H.; Jones, A.; Stark, L.: Dynamics of head movement trajectories: main sequence relationship. Expl Neurol. *71:* 76–91 (1981).

Prof. R. Schmid, Dipartimento di Informatica e Sistemistica,
Università di Pavia, Via Abbiategrasso 209, I-27100 Pavia (Italy)

Adv. Oto-Rhino-Laryng., vol. 41, pp. 95–97 (Karger, Basel 1988)

Distribution of Retinal Ganglion Cells Projecting into the Nucleus of the Optic Tract in Rat

Tamotu Urushibata, Isao Kato, Tomoyuki Okada, Isamu Takeyama

Department of Otolaryngology, St. Marianna University School of Medicine, Kawasaki, Japan

Recent neurophysiological studies have disclosed that the nucleus of the optic tract (NOT) in the pretectum is the first relay station responsible for horizontal optokinetic nystagmus (OKN) both in non-foveal [1–3] and foveal animals [4]. However, it is still open to discussion as to from what parts of the retina and what kinds of retinal ganglion cells project their fibers into the NOT. In the present study, horse-radish peroxidase conjugated with wheat-germ agglutin (WGA-HRP) was injected into the NOT of rats. The retinas and injection sites were processed for the histochemical demonstration of WGA-HRP in order to investigate the distribution of the retinal ganglion cells projecting into the NOT.

Material and Methods

Wistar rats (250–270 g) were anesthetized with intraperitoneal injection of pentobarbital sodium (20 mg/kg). A 10% solution of WGA-HRP was injected into the NOT through a glass micropipette. After a survival time of 48 h, the animals were reanesthetized and perfused with 0.9% saline followed by fixation. Injection sites of the brain and the retina were processed for histochemical demonstration of WGA-HRP by tetramethyl benzidine protocol and Hanker Yeats' method.

Results

The injection site was identified as dark-brown color in and around the NOT extending to adjacent structures. For this reason, the superior colliculus (SC) and the dorsolateral geniculate body (dLGB) were examined as controls in search of any differences among them. The soma size of these cells varied

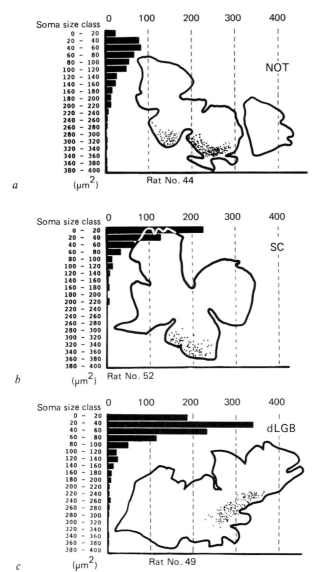

Fig. 1. a–c Areas of labeled cells in the retina ipsilateral to each injection site. The upper drawing represents NOT (*a*); the middle, SC (*b*); the lower, dLGB (*c*). Every dot indicates a labeled cell. The histograms show the frequency distribution of cell body sizes. Ordinate: Soma size class (each range represents 20 μm^2). Abscissa: Numbers of labeled cells per class. Large cells were defined as cells of about 30 μm diameter; medium-sized cells, about 15 μm diameter; small cells, about 5 μm diameter. Small and medium-sized cells project into the NOT (*a*), rather small-sized cells project into the SC (*b*) and the dLGB (*c*).

depending upon whether the dendrites of the cells were stained or not. Therefore, soma areas of labeled cells were at first photographed 250 times actual size as large as they are and then measured by using a device in order to distinguish labeled cells from each other in greater detail. After WGA-HRP injection in the NOT, the labeled cells were observed in the whole area of the retina contralateral to the injection site. However, no relationship could be seen between soma sizes and regions of the retina. This relationship was identical whether WGA-HRP was injected into the SC or the dLGB close to the NOT. However, judging from the frequency distribution of soma sizes, large-sized cells were prevalent in the dLGB, medium-sized cells in the SC, and small-sized cells in the NOT. Labeled cells were located only in the ventral region of the retina ipsilateral to the injection site. Furthermore, cell density in the ventral region of the retina differed in areas ipsilateral and contralateral to the injection site in the NOT, being about 4 times greater in the retina ipsilateral to the injection site (fig. 1).

Summary

The present study indicates that visual signals responsible for OKN are conducted through the retinal ganglion cells mainly contralaterally, and only in the ventral region of the retina ipsilateral to the injection site. The retinal ganglion cells projecting into the NOT ipsilateral to the injection site were identified as small- and medium-sized cells in the rat. The density of the ventral ganglion cells of the retina contralateral to the injection site was lower than that in any other regions of the retina except for the dorsal region of the retina, and the density of the ventral ganglion cells ipsilateral to the injection site was about 4 times greater than that on the contralateral side. This finding requires physiological investigation in the future.

References

1   Collewijin, H.: Direction-selective units in the rabbit's nucleus of the optic tract. Brain Res. *100:* 489–508 (1975).
2   Hoffmann, K.-P.; Schoppmann, A.: Retinal input to direction-selective cells in the nucleus tractus opticus of the cat. Brain Res. *99:* 359–366 (1975).
3   Precht, W.; Strata, P.: On the pathway mediating optokinetic responses in vestibular nuclear neurons. Neuroscience *5:* 777–787 (1980).
4   Kato, I.; et al.: Role of nucleus of the optic tract in monkeys in relation to optokinetic nystagmus. Brain Res. *364:* 12–22 (1986).

T. Urushibata, MD, Department of Otolaryngology, St. Marianna University School of Medicine 2-16-1, Sugao, Miyamae-ku, 213 Kawasaki (Japan)

Adv. Oto-Rhino-Laryng., vol. 41, pp. 98–103 (Karger, Basel 1988)

Effects of Pretectal Lesions in Monkeys on Two Components of Optokinetic Nystagmus

Takao Ikarashi[a], *Isao Kato*[b], *Koji Harada*[a], *Tomohiko Hasegawa*[a], *Yoshio Koike*[a]

[a]Department of Otolaryngology, Yamagata University School of Medicine, Yamagata; [b]Department of Otolaryngology, St. Marianna University School of Medicine, Kanagawa, Japan

Introduction

Recent neurophysiological studies have disclosed that the nucleus of the optic tract (NOT) is the sensorimotor link between the retina and premotor structures in the pathway mediating the optokinetic reflex in rats, rabbits, cats and monkeys.

Generally, in monkeys, optokinetic nystagmus (OKN) can be divided into two components: an initial rapid and slower rise in slow phase OKN velocity in response to a constant velocity stimulus [1]. A rapid rise in the slow phase OKN velocity is thought to be mediated through the visual cortex and the flocculus may reflect the contribution of the pursuit system. A slower rise in slow phase OKN velocity reflects activation of a velocity storage mechanism and is associated with production of optokinetic after-nystagmus (OKAN) that is shared in common with the vestibular system [3].

We have clarified the role of the NOT in the fascicularis monkeys in the generation of OKN [2]. This monkey, however, does not show any initial rapid rise during optokinetic stimulation.

In the present experiments, the fuscata monkey, that is said to hold an initial rapid rise during the step-induced optokinetic stimulation, was investigated by making a lesion in the pretectum.

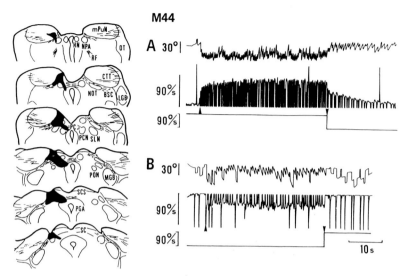

Fig. 1. Histological presentation of left pretectal lesions of monkey 44 (left side). Lesion sites are filled with black. Sections are rostrocaudal from above to below. Effects of left pretectal lesions on OKN and OKAN in monkey 44 (right side). The upper trace in each series is DC-EOG during OK stimulation to the right *(A)* and to the left *(B)*. The second trace in *A* and *B* shows slow-phase velocity. The bottom trace in *A* and *B* shows stimulus velocity.

Materials and Methods

Ten fuscata monkeys were used in the present experiment. Eye movements were recorded with DC-EOG. The EOG was differentiated by amplifiers with a 0.03 second time constant and rectified to obtain the velocity of the slow phase of nystagmus. After preoperative control, the left anterolateral border of the superior colliculus was destroyed by electrolytical method or the use of 0.01% kainic acid. Follow-up studies started from the 7th postoperative day onward at about one-week intervals.

After long-term observation of the postoperative course, the brain of the animal was perfused with physiological saline and 10% formalin through the left ventricle. The extent of the lesion was checked by paraffin section stained with Klüver-Barrera.

Results

Extent of Lesions

According to the extent of the lesion, monkeys were classified into three groups. (1) Representative histological drawing obtained from monkey 44 in the first group is shown in figure 1. The lesions involved totally the NOT in

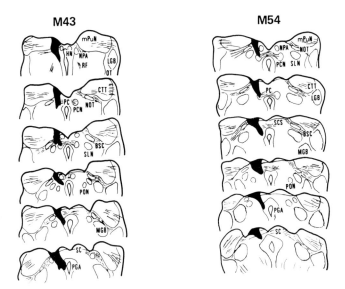

Fig. 2. Histological presentation of left medial pretectal lesions of monkeys 43 (left) and 54 (right). The nuclei of the posterior commissure are damaged in both animals.

the lateral part of the pretectum from the rostral part to the caudal part and the nucleus of the posterior commissure partially in the medial part of the pretectum. (2) Representative histological drawings obtained from monkeys 43 and 54 who were classified in the second group are shown in figure 2. In monkey 43, destroyed electrolytically, and monkey 54, destroyed by the use of 0.1% kainic acid, the former involved the medial part of the pretectum including the nucleus of the posterior commissure. The latter involved the same area in monkey 43. (3) Representative histological drawings were obtained from monkeys 45 and 50 (fig. 3), who were classified in the third group. Chemically produced lesions in monkey 45 involved the lateral part in the left pretectum including the NOT. In monkey 50, the same lesions were observed as in monkey 45. Both chemically and electrolytically produced lesions involved the lateral part of the pretectum including the NOT.

Effects of Lesions on OKN and OKAN

In monkey 44, who was classified in the first group, an initial rapid rise of slow phase velocity toward the lesion side was reduced in 50% after operation; a slower rise and OKAN were severely impaired (fig. 1).

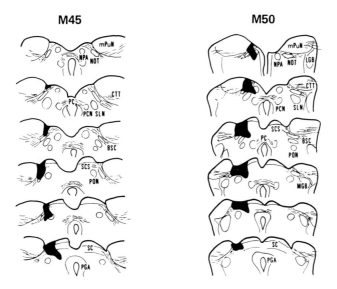

Fig. 3. Histological presentation of left lateral pretectal lesions including NOT of monkeys 45 (left) and 50 (right).

In monkey 43, with electrolytically produced lesions in the second group, the initial rapid rise toward the lesion side was severely impaired, while in monkey 54, with chemically produced lesions, the initial rapid rise showed a normal pattern (fig. 4).

In monkeys 45 and 50, who were classified in the third group, in spite of the difference in destruction methods, the slower rise of slow phase velocity of OKN toward the lesion side was impaired and OKAN was also impaired, but initial rapid rise was not impaired (fig. 5).

In other visually induced eye movements, such as pursuit, saccadic eye movements were quantitatively normal and gaze holding was also perfect, as reported in fascicularis monkeys [2].

Discussion

Lesions in the lateral pretectum of the first and third groups (NOT lesion) had drastic and selective effects upon reducing the slower rise, and

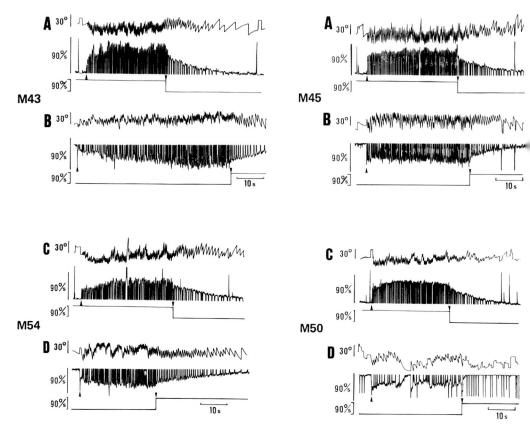

Fig. 4. Effects of left medial pretectal lesions on OKN and OKAN of monkeys 43 (above) and 54 (below). The same symbols and layout as in figure 1 are used.

Fig. 5. Effects of left pretectal lesions on OKN and OKAN of monkeys 45 (above) and 50 (below). The same symbols and layout as in figure 1 are used.

OKAN in the slow phase velocity toward the lesion side. Lesions in the medial pretectum, by electrolytical destruction of the first and second groups, had selective effects upon reducing an initial rapid rise in slow phase velocity toward the lesion side. The present experiment demonstrated, in the lesion of the lateral pretectum, a slower rise and OKAN were impaired, but VOR showed a normal pattern, except for vestibular habituation of repeated testing.

Therefore, this study indicates that the NOT plays an important role for elicitation of OKN and OKAN in the monkey as in other species. NOT will take a position for driving the velocity storage integrator. From our experimental results, the dynamics in charge of the velocity storage mechanism are selectively influenced by the destruction of the NOT. Moreover, the fiber of passage through the medial part of the pretectum will also influence the occurrence of the initial rapid rise.

References

1   Cohen, B.; Matsuo, V.; Raphan, T.: Quantitative analysis of the velocity characteristics of optokinetic nystagmus and optokinetic after-nystagmus. J. Physiol. *270:* 321–344 (1977).
2   Kato, I.; Harada, K.; Hasegawa, T.; Ikarashi, T.; Koike, Y.; Kawasaki, T.: Role of the nucleus of the optic tract in monkeys in relation to optokinetic nystagmus. Brain Res. *364:* 12–22 (1986).
3   Robinson, D.A.: Control of eye movements; in Handbook of physiology. The nervous system. Am. Physiol. Soc., Bethesda 1981, sect. 1, vol. 2, pp. 1275–1320.

Takao Ikarashi, MD, Department of Otolaryngology,
Yamagata University School of Medicine, Yamagata 990-23 (Japan)

Adv. Oto-Rhino-Laryng., vol. 41, pp. 104–108 (Karger, Basel 1988)

Abnormalities of Visually Induced Eye Movements in Thalamic Lesions

Tadashi Nakamura[a], *Isao Kato*[b], *Ryoji Kanayama*[a], *Yoshio Koike*[a]

[a] Department of Otolaryngology, Yamagata University School of Medicine, Zao-Iida, Yamagata; [b] Department of Otolaryngology, St. Marianna University School of Medicine, Miyamae, Kanagawa, Japan

Introduction

The thalamus consists of many nuclei that act as a relay and integrating station in the major neural system. Although various oculomotor abnormalities have been observed in the thalamic hemorrhage, the exact role of the thalamus in the eye movement control still remains unclear. In this report, a quantitative analysis of the optokinetic nystagmus (OKN) and smooth pursuit eye movement was performed using a computer system in 18 patients with thalamic hemorrhage.

Materials and Methods

Eighteen patients with thalamic hemorrhage accurately located by computer tomography (CT) were selected for the present study. The patients had normal visual field and no horizontal and vertical tonic eye deviations. OKN were induced by the rotating stripes at a constant velocity of 30, 40, 50 and 60 °/s in both directions. For smooth pursuit, the patients were asked to track a small dot moving in a sinusoidal pattern at a frequency of 0.3 Hz and an amplitude of 20°. The analog data of the eye position was digitized at a rate of 200 samples/s through a 12-bit analog-digital converter. The gain of the slow-phase velocity of OKN (spv-OKN) was computed by dividing the average of the spv-OKN by the stimulus velocity, and the pursuit gain was measured by the ratio of the peak eye velocity, after removal of corrective saccades from the tracing, to the peak target velocity.

Table I. The findings of the slow-phase velocity of OKN and smooth pursuit

Case no.	ETT		OKN	
	lesion side	intact side	lesion side	intact side
Group A				
1–3	–	–	–	–
Group B				
4–6	–	–	+	–
7, 8	–	–	+++	+
9, 10	–	–	++	+
Group C				
11	+	–	+	–
12	++	+	+++	++
13	++	–	+++	–
14	+	+	+	+
15	++	++	++	++
16–18	++	++	+++	+++

– = Normal; + = slightly impaired; ++ = moderately impaired; +++ = severely impaired; ETT = eye tracking test.

Results

A previous study indicated that in normal subjects the gain of the spv-OKN was more than 0.8 at stimulus velocity less than 60 °/s and the pursuit gain was more than 0.8 [8]. The results of this study are shown in table I. The gain of the spv-OKN reduced markedly compared with normal limits in 15 patients. Although 5 patients had impaired OKN in both directions, the asymmetry of OKN impairment was observed in 10 patients in whom OKN, when directed toward the lesion side, was impaired more than when directed toward the intact side. Eight of 18 patients had impaired smooth pursuit, and the pursuit gain reduced remarkably when the target moved toward the lesion side in 4 patients.

Judging from impairment of the spv-OKN and smooth pursuit in 18 patients, three groups could be classified: (group A) the gain of the spv-OKN and smooth pursuit are within normal range; (group B) the gain of the spv-OKN reduced markedly but pursuit gain remains normal; (group C) both the spv-OKN and smooth pursuit are impaired.

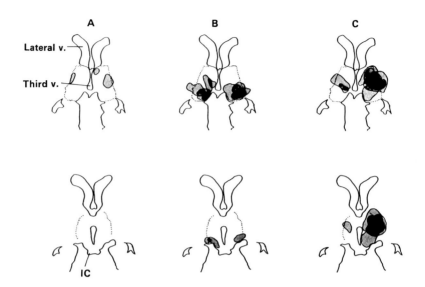

Fig. 1. The illustration of the lesions in groups A–C. The shaded area indicates a high density mass consisting of blood on CT scan data. IC = Inferior colliculus.

Figure 1 illustrates the lesions based on the CT scan data. The cases of group A had the smallest lesions in this study, which involved the limited anterior thalamus without involvements of the posterior thalamus and midbrain (fig. 1A). The lesions in group B mainly involved the posterior area of the thalamus but with sparing of the anterior area of the thalamus (fig. 1B). The cases of group C had the largest lesions among all the patients with extensive involvements of the thalamus and extended to the midbrain (fig. 1C).

Discussion

In the present study, the spv-OKN was extremely limited in 15 patients and 8 patients had asymmetrical impairments of OKN. We previously reported that in the patients who had unilateral lesions in the midbrain, the cerebellum and the tegmentum of the pontine base, the spv-OKN was more decreased when the stripes rotated toward the lesion side [6]. Whereas there is a clinical report of the impairment of OKN and smooth pursuit in parietal lobe lesions, in which the spv-OKN was more impaired when the stripes moved toward the lesion side [1]. It was reported that the low-gain pursuit when directed toward the damaged side was recognized in a small lesion of the posterior thalamus [2].

There are many experimental studies concerning the pathway of OKN and smooth pursuit. OKN was almost abolished in cats with the lesions in the nucleus of the optic tract (NOT) [7] and the nucleus reticularis tegmenti pontis (NRTP) [4]. Thus, NOT acts as the first relay station in the optokinetic pathway, and there are crucial links between NOT and NRTP in this pathway [7]. Whereas the parietal cortex was observed to project to the lateral NRTP, the descending fibers for the frontal and parietal eye field probably track in close proximity at the level of the thalamus [5]. From these studies, the lesions of the posterior thalamus presumably disrupt this pathway, resulting in the OKN impairment.

The OKN was impaired but with normal pursuit gain the evidence suggests that there are two separate pathways between OKN and smooth pursuit. This indicates that two such types of eye movements share the same pathway in the brain stem [8]. Another investigation, however, revealed that OKN was completely abolished despite the normal pursuit gain in the lesions of NOT in monkeys [3]. Many investigators reported that there are two separate pathways, i.e. cortical and subcortical, which are used for the generation of OKN induced by a surrounding optokinetic stimulus because of the stimulation of both the fovea and retina [1, 8]. The result in the cases of group B suggests that these findings result from the disruption of the only subcortical pathway of OKN. The distinction between cortical and subcortical OKN, however, still remains unclear and this problem will be clarified in the near future.

References

1   Baloh, R.W.; Yee, R.D.; Honrubia, V.: Optokinetic nystagmus and parietal lobe lesions. Ann. Neurol. *7:* 269–276 (1980).
2   Brigell, M.; Babikian, V.; Goodwin, J.A.: Hypometric saccades and low-gain pursuit resulting from a thalamic hemorrhage. Ann. Neurol. *15:* 374–378 (1984).
3   Kato, I.; Harada, K.; Hasegawa, T.; et al.: Role of the nucleus of the optic tract in monkeys in relation to optokinetic nystagmus. Brain Res. *364:* 12–22 (1986).
4   Kato, I.; Harada, K.; Nakamura, T.; et al.: Role of the nucleus reticularis tegmenti pontis on visually induced eye movements. Expl Neurol. *781:* 503–516 (1982).
5   Leichnetz, G.R.; Smith, D.J.; Spencer, R.F.: Cortical projection to the paramedian tegmental and basilar pons in the monkey. J. comp. Neurol. *228:* 388–408 (1984).

6 Nakamura, T.; Kato, I.; Kanayama, R.; et al.: Computer analysis of optokinetic nystagmus for clinical usefulness. Auris Nasus Larynx *13:* suppl. 11, pp. 97–103 (1986).
7 Precht, W.: Visual-vestibular interaction in vestibular neurons: functional pathway organization. Ann. N.Y. Acad. Sci. *374:* 230–248 (1981).
8 Yee, R.D.; Baloh, R.D.; Honrubia, et al.: Slow build-up of optokinetic nystagmus associated with downbeat nystagmus. Investve Ophthal. vis. Sci. *18:* 622–629 (1979).

Tadashi Nakamura, MD, Department of Otolaryngology,
Yamagata University School of Medicine, Zao-Iida, Yamagata 990-23 (Japan)

Adv. Oto-Rhino-Laryng., vol. 41, pp. 109–115 (Karger, Basel 1988)

A Comparison between Smooth Pursuit and Visual Suppression[1]

L.M. Ödkvist, J. Thell, B. Larsby

Department of Otolaryngology, University Hospital, Linköping, Sweden

The smooth pursuit system stabilizes a moving target on the fovea by producing eye velocity that closely matches target velocity. The visual suppression system inhibits or cancels the vestibulo-ocular reflex (VOR) when the head movements do not coincide with the visual target movements. An earlier theory concerning the visual suppression of vestibular nystagmus and smooth ocular pursuit has been that they use the same neuronal structures or even that they are the same system. Later reports have indicated that the smooth pursuit and visual suppression systems have similar characteristics but are not the same system.

The present investigation reports findings from 24 patients with pathology in the smooth pursuit system and/or pathology in the visual suppression system. They were compared to normals.

Material

Twenty-four consecutive patients with pathology in the smooth pursuit and/or the visual suppression mechanisms were included in the study. The age range was 15–77 years (mean 53; SD = 16). The diagnoses were cerebellar tumour, infarction or hyperplasia (5 cases), arterial loop syndrome (3 cases), processes influencing the brain stem (5 cases), primary fibromyalgia (5 cases), Parkinson's disease (1 case), cerebral metastasis (1 case), unknown CNS cause (4 cases).

The patients were compared to 15 healthy volunteers in the age range 22–56 years (mean 34; SD = 8). None of these volunteers had any history of ocular or oculomotor dysfunction. All subjects had good visual acuity either normally or after correction.

[1] This study was supported by the Medical Research Council.

Methods

The patients and the test persons were investigated with the routine electronystag-mography (ENG) procedure. A visual suppression test and a smooth pursuit test were added.

Smooth Pursuit Test

The pursuit target stimulus was a laser dot on the wall moved by a computerized program in either a sinusoidal frequency sweep or in a pseudorandomized pattern, the frequencies used being 0.25–2.0 Hz. The horizontal eye movements in response to the stimulation were recorded by electro-oculography (EOG). The eye signal was amplified, A/D-converted and fed to a desk-top computer for analysis. A signal of the target motion was also A/D-converted and fed to the computer. Each stimulation trial had a duration of 40 s. The maximum target velocity was kept constant at 20 or 40 °/s in the different runs.

Visual Suppression Test

The visual suppression test was performed while the patient was situated in the rotatory chair. The moving pattern was identical to the one used in the smooth pursuit test. The test was performed in 40-second trials in the light. The patients were instructed to fixate a dot on a frame mounted on the chair and thus all the time being directly in front of the eyes. EOG was performed. The head movements (chair movements) were recorded by an angular rate sensor attached to a bite board. The eye and head movement signals during the 40-second period were fed into a computer for analysis.

Data Analysis

The eye position signal and the target position signal/head position signal were A/D-converted at a sampling frequency of 100 Hz and then stored on floppy disks. From the pursuit eye movement signal, containing both saccades and smooth components, a cumulative slow eye movement curve was constructed by removal of saccades and artefacts. The eye position signal and the target position signal were then differentiated to give velocity values. The head movement rate sensor gives the velocity values without differentiation. The fast Fourier transform and power spectrum analysis techniques were used to calculate the gain (eye velocity/target velocity or head velocity) and phase (the temporal relationship between the eye velocity and target velocity or head velocity) as a function of stimulation frequency both for the composite and the smooth eye movement curves [1–3]. Statistical analysis between trials was performed using Student's t-test. In many patients an asymmetry in the cumulative edited eye movement curve appeared. It was denounced a linear DC-trend and expressed in degrees per second.

Results

The normal subjects showed pursuit movements with a gain close to 1 at low frequencies in the sinusoidal frequency sweep stimulation test. The gain decreased with increasing stimulation frequency. For the same sinusoidal

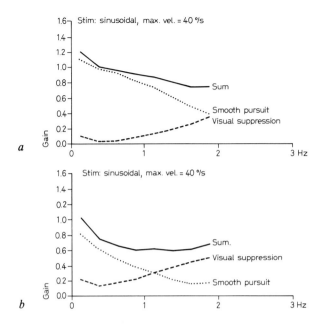

Fig. 1. In the broad frequency tests the smooth pursuit gain (····) and the visual suppression gain (----) are given as a function of stimulus frequency. The sum of the gain values for each frequency is given by the unbroken line (Sum). *a* Mean values from 15 normals and *b* from 24 patients with CNS disturbance. Gain=Eye velocity/stimulus velocity.

frequency sweep stimulation pattern the visual suppression was very effective for low frequencies with a gain close to 0. For increasing frequencies the visual suppression diminished and gain increased (fig. 1).

In the patients many variations were present. As a group the patients showed a decreased smooth pursuit gain and a decreased visual suppression ability (fig. 1, lower part), the group values being significantly different ($p > 0.01$) from the values in the normals.

The influence of prediction of the smooth pursuit gain was studied by comparing the smooth pursuit gain for sinusoidal and pseudorandomized stimulation (fig. 2). The gain when a pseudorandomized stimulus was used was considerably lower in comparison to smooth pursuit. However,

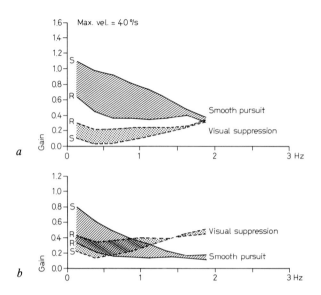

Fig. 2. The smooth pursuit gain decreased when a randomized stimulus pattern was used (R) as compared to the gain for a sinusoidal pattern (S). The striped area shows the decrease. The visual suppression gain increased when the stimulus was changed from sinusoidal (S) to randomized (R). The dotted area shows the change. *a* 15 normals; *b* 24 patients.

with visual suppression the gain increased. The visual suppression ability proved to be less dependent on the stimulus pattern (fig. 2). The visual suppression ability in the patient group seemed also less dependent upon stimulus pattern than the pursuit ability in the patient group (fig. 2, lower part).

The asymmetry in the visual suppression test and the pursuit test as it appears in the DC trend was calculated. For sinusoidal stimulation there was no difference between the pursuit trend and the visual suppression trend in normals, but for the patient group, however, there was a significant difference ($p < 0.10$). For randomized stimulation there was no trend difference between the pursuit test and the visual suppression test either in normals or in the patient group. When normals were compared to patients in the sinusoidal visual suppression test there was a significant ($p > 0.05$) difference in trend values. The normals' and the patients' trend in the pursuit test were significantly different for the sinusoidal as well as for the randomized stimulation (p>0.10). In the randomized visual suppression test, however, there was no trend difference between normals and patients.

Eleven patients had a pathological smooth pursuit test, 13 patients had pathology in the pursuit test as well as in the visual suppression test but in the series no patient appeared who had pathology in the visual suppression test alone.

Discussion

The visual suppression and the smooth pursuit system have the same task of keeping the visual target on the fovea. The conditions for the two systems are, however, somewhat different as the pursuit system mainly functions when the visual surrounding is in movement and the visual suppression system is in action when the VOR is stimulated by head movements. The smooth pursuit ability as measured by the velocity gain seems to decrease with increasing frequency [3]. The visual suppression ability decreases with increasing frequency possibly mainly due to the increasing importance of VOR with increasing frequency [2, 4-6]. Leigh et al. [7] found that in normal subjects VOR cancellation was more effective than what would have been predicted from their smooth pursuit performance. This finding is in accordance with results reported by McKinley and Petersen [8] using non-predictable stimuli. The present investigation in a consecutive series of patients describes patients with pathology in the visual suppression system as well as in the smooth pursuit system and also patients with pathology only in the smooth pursuit system. There appeared, however, no patients with pathology in the visual suppression system alone. This is not in accordance with the material presented by Chambers and Gresty [9], who described patients even with this single feature. Chambers and Gresty [9], however, are using a totally different stimulation system and calculation parameters using fixed frequency stimulation and using the peak slow eye movement velocity as the parameter.

The fact that smooth pursuit gain is not mirroring the visual suppression gain and the higher influence of randomization on the smooth pursuit gain compared to the influence on the visual suppression gain indicates that the smooth pursuit system and the visual suppression system are not identical (fig. 2). If they had been identical the sum of the smooth pursuit gain and the visual suppression gain would have been equal to 1 (fig. 1).

The trend difference pattern also indicates that the two systems are different or at least are not totally identical. If they were identical an asymmetry in the pursuit test would be mirrored by an asymmetry in the visual suppression ability.

The effect of age has to be taken into consideration as there was a mean age difference between the patient group and the normals. The decrease in pursuit and visual suppression ability does not seem to deteriorate due to age until after 65 or 70 years of age, however [3].

The clinical test procedure presented in this study is easy to perform and quantifies visual tracking ability as well as visual suppression ability over a wide frequency range [3, 10]. The advantage with the present setup is that the stimulus pattern concerning frequency and velocity are identical for the two tests. The key point for both systems seems to be the cerebellar flocculus [9]. In what parts of the CNS the two mechanisms differ is yet to be discovered.

Conclusion

It may be concluded that testing the smooth pursuit ability and the visual suppression function is clinically useful as a defect in any of those systems is a certain evidence for CNS pathology, usually in the posterior fossa.

References

1   Mairy, J.L.: The vestibular system and human dynamic space orientation. NASA CR-628 Washington 1966.
2   Larsby, B.; Tomlinson, R.D.; Schwarz, D.W.S.; Istl, Y.; Fredrickson, J.M. Quantification of the vestibulo-ocular reflex and visual-vestibular interaction for the purpose of clinical diagnosis. Med. biol. Eng. Comp. 20: 99–107 (1982).
3   Larsby, B., Thell, J.; Möller, C.; Ödkvist, L.: The effect of stimulus predictability and age on human tracking eye movements. Acta oto-lar. 105: 21–30 (1988).
4   Hydén, D.; Larsby, B.; Möller, C.; Ödkvist, L.M.; Ekvall, L.: Rotatory and caloric findings in patients with acoustic neuromas; in Graham, Kimink, The vestibular system. Neurophysiologic and clinical research, pp. 379-385 (Raven Press, New York 1987).
5   Larsby, B.; Hydén, D.; Ödkvist, L.M.: Gain and phase characteristics of compensatory eye movements in light and darkness. A study with a broad frequency band rotatory test. Acta oto-lar. 97: 223-234 (1984).
6   Ödkvist, L.M.; Möller, C.; Larsby, B.; Hydén, D.: Vestibular compensation measured by the broad frequency band rotatory test; in Graham, Kimink, The vestibular system. Neurophysiologic and clinical research, pp. 313–318 (Raven Press, New York 1987).

7   Leigh, R.J.; Sharpe, J.A.; Ranalli, P.J.; Hamid, M.A.; Thurston, S.E.: Comparison of smooth pursuit and combined eye head tracking in normal subjects with deficient labyrinthine function. Soc. Neurosci. Abstr. *11:* 1083 (1985).
8   McKinley, P.A.; Petersen, B.W.: Voluntary modulation of the vestibulo-ocular reflex by mental effort in darkness. Exp. Brain Res. *60:* 454-464 (1985).
9   Chambers, B.R.; Gresty, M.A.: The relationship between disordered pursuit and vestibulo-ocular reflex suppression. J. Neurol. Neurosurg. Psychiat. *46:* 61-66 (1983).
10 Larsby, B.; Thell, J.; Ödkvist, L.M.: A computerized smooth pursuit test; in Claussen, Kirtane, Vertigo, nausea, tinnitus and hearing loss in cadiovascular disease, pp. 313–318 (Elsevier, Amsterdam 1986).

Lars M. Ödkvist, MD, Department Otolaryngology, University Hospital,
S-581 85 Linköping (Sweden)

Adv. Oto-Rhino-Laryng., vol. 41, pp. 116–117 (Karger, Basel 1988)

Some Mechanisms in the Predictive Control of Smooth Pursuit Eye Movements

A.W. Kornhuber, R. Jürgens, W. Becker

Sektion Neurophysiologie, Universität Ulm, Ulm, FRG

Smooth pursuit eye movements (SPEM) do not just follow a moving target. It has been shown that the oculomotor system is capable of tracking periodic stimuli with zero latency in spite of the inevitable delays in the visual system. Is SPEM in such a situation then generated exclusively by predictive mechanisms without the intervention of retinal error signals? We addressed this question with a series of experiments in which we manipulated the retinal error signals by the open-loop method (eye position is electronically added to target position). Eye movements were recorded by a scleral search coil.

Subjects track a sinusoidally moving target of, say, 0.5 Hz, thus SPEM is perfectly in phase with the target, except for a small superimposed oscillation of about 3 Hz, which creates a corresponding error signal. When the target is suddenly stabilized on the fovea (by switching to the OL regime), the oscillation disappears, while the basic 0.5 Hz SPEM vanishes only slowly (within 5–10 s) and decreases gradually its frequency. This demonstrates that even zero latency tracking requires a retinal error signal and cannot be explained solely by prediction.

Several factors were identified which may contribute to the predictive component of SPEM:

(1) With retinal position or velocity errors held constant (again by using the OL regime), a relationship between eye position, eye velocity and eye acceleration can be shown: the faster the eye travels towards the limits of expected eccentricity [$\pm 25°$] (or eye's motility range), the faster the acceleration is reduced, and finally reversed, in order to stop SPEM; this relation between current velocity and acceleration is accentuated as the expected current eye position draws closer to limits. In tracking of periodic targets this

is tantamount to a pseudoprediction of the inevitable turnaround of the target movement.

(2) An important mechanism is the subject's 'internal synchronization' to the time frame underlying the target movement. When subjects track a random sequence of to and fro ramps with different velocities (5–20 °/s) but constant intervals between successive ramps, they anticipate the onset of the next ramp starting their movement in synchrony with, or even slightly prior to, the onset of the ramp. This becomes particularly clear when, instead of starting the next ramp movement, the target is unexpectedly stabilized on the fovea. In this situation subjects initiate nonetheless a 'response' which is often indistinguishable from responses to normal 5 °/s ramps, but far smaller in amplitude than the average response.

A.W. Kornhuber, MD, Sektion Neurophysiologie, Universität Ulm,
D–7900 Ulm (FRG)

Adv. Oto-Rhino-Laryng., vol. 41, pp. 118–121 (Karger, Basel 1988)

Normal Predictive Function in Smooth Pursuit

Naoki Ohashi, Yukio Watanabe, Kanemasa Mizukoshi, Hatuo Ino

Department of Otolaryngology, Faculty of Medicine,
Toyama Medical and Pharmaceutical University, Toyama, Japan

Introduction

It is believed that the predictive function in smooth pursuit makes a contribution to keep the eye movement smooth. However, previous investigations [1–3] on the predictive function have not concluded which attribute of the target movement they were mainly focused on, particularly the relationship between the attributes and the prediction. Therefore, we developed a target movement in which the direction of the sinusoidal wave is the only variance. Five parameters were obtained and the frequency analysis was performed between the predictive and nonpredictive portions.

Materials and Methods

Twenty-three healthy volunteers, collected as the normal subjects, sat in the center of a target projection screen having a diameter of 1.5 m. The target movement (random sinusoidal wave) was developed with an 8-bit microcomputer (CBM 8032) by the authors. The random sinusoidal wave (fig. 1) contains 40 half sinusoidal waves. The basic frequency of the random sinusoidal wave can be selected from one of 5 frequencies (0.6, 0.8, 1.0, 1.2 and 1.4 Hz). The eye movements and target movements (random sinusoidal wave) were converted to the digital value with a 12-bit A/D converter at 10-ms intervals. Five parameters — amplitude gain, retinal error velocity (abbreviated as REV), velocity gain, acceleration gain and phase lag — were calculated. The frequency analysis (by the FFT method) was performed on target movements and eye movements to obtain the power spectrum. The subtraction of the power spectrum of target movements from that of eye movements was obtained. The calculation was performed both in the predictive and nonpredictive portions.

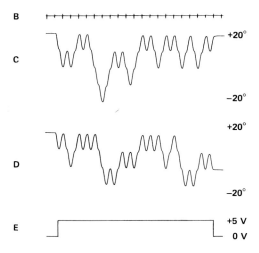

Fig. 1. The random sinusoidal wave moves in the range of +(right)20° and –(left)20°. The basic frequency of the original sinusoidal wave is selected from one of 5 frequencies (0.6, 0.8, 1.0, 1.2 and 1.4 Hz). The amplitude of the original sinusoidal wave is 5°.

Results

As the frequency of the random sinusoidal wave increases from 0.6 Hz, phase lag gradually increases in both the predictive and nonpredictive portions. Further, in higher frequencies above 1.2 Hz there is a significant difference (t-test $p < 0.01$) between the predictive and nonpredictive portions (fig. 2). However, there were no significant differences between the predictive and nonpredictive portions in the other 4 parameters. The subtraction of the power spectra becomes negative in the range from 0.8 to 2.4 Hz. However, the subtraction of the power spectra above 2.7 Hz is significantly (t-test $p < 0.01$) higher in the predictive portions than in the nonpredictive portions in the basic frequencies from 0.6 to 1.4 Hz (fig. 3).

Discussion

The studies of the predictive function in smooth pursuit have been performed by several investigators. The present result was consistent with the previous reports that the phase lag was kept at a minimum if the target

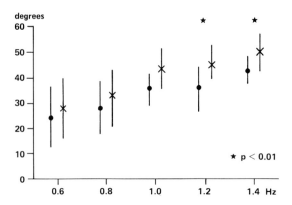

Fig. 2. Phase lag (mean ± SD) obtained from 23 normal subjects is presented as a function of the basic frequency. Dots and Xs are the means of phase lag in the predictive and nonpredictive portions, respectively. The significant differences (t-test p <0.01) were noted in higher frequencies above 1.2 Hz.

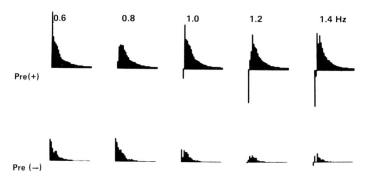

Fig. 3. The subtraction of the power spectra of target movements from those of eye movements were performed in 9 normal subjects. Pre (+) and pre (—) mean the predictive and nonpredictive portions, respectively. The frequency range of the FFT is from 0.8 to 25.0 Hz. The differences between two portions (predictive and nonpredictive) are significant above 2.7 Hz in 5 basic frequencies. The power spectra from 0.0 to 0.4 Hz were influenced from the base line drift so those power spectra were excluded from this figure.

movement is predictive. The fact that the power spectra in the range above 2.7 Hz was significantly higher in the predictive portion may lead to the following hypothesis: that is, the predictor in the central nervous system calculates the power spectrum of the target movement [4–6]. And the inverse FFT is disposed simultaneously to maintain the phase at a minimum and consequently sustain the ongoing smooth pursuit.

Conclusion

We have developed a random sinusoidal wave to investigate the predictive function in smooth pursuit. The predictive function in smooth pursuit in normal subjects serves the function of maintaining the phase at a minimum. The higher power spectrum of the eye movements sustains the ongoing smooth pursuit.

References

1   Dollas, P.J.; Jones, R.W.: Learning behavior of the eye fixation control system. IEEE Trans. automat. Control *July*: 218–227 (1962).
2   Stark, L.; Vossius, G.; Young, L.R.: Predictive control of eye tracking movements. IRE Trans. hum. Fact. Electron. *Sept.:* 52–57 (1962).
3   Michael, J.A.; Jones, G.M.: Dependence of visual tracking capability upon stimulus predictability. Vision Res. *6:* 707–716 (1966).
4   Ohashi, N.; Watanabe, Y.; Mizukoshi, K.; Kobayashi, H.: Quantitative measurement of smooth pursuit using the continuously changing sinusoidal wave in normal subjects. ORL *47:* 49–56 (1985).
5   Ohashi, N.; Watanabe, Y.; Mizukoshi, K.; Kobayashi, H.: Quantitative comparison between saccadic and ataxic pursuits. Acta oto-lar. *101:* 200–206 (1986).
6   Ohashi. N.; Watanabe, Y.; Mizukoshi, K.: Prediction in smooth pursuit. Acta oto-lar. *103:* 131–136 (1987).

Naoki Ohashi, MD, Department of Otolaryngology, Faculty of Medicine, Toyama Medical and Pharmaceutical University, Toyama (Japan)

Adv. Oto-Rhino-Laryng., vol. 41, pp. 122–126 (Karger, Basel 1988)

Saccadic Eye Movements Induced by Directional Hearing Stimuli

Dethard Nagel, W. Gdynia

ENT Department, University Clinic of Ulm
(Head Prof. Dr. Reinhard Pfalz), Ulm, FRG

Introduction

To a human with physiological stereophonic hearing, noise usually has directional information associated with it. This impression is created through differences in intensity, transmission delays and phase shifts. The directional auditory stimulus, modulated by the relative attentiveness of the listener, causes certain sensory and motion responses. Typically the eyes respond with several quick scanning movements towards the perceived source of the noise (aiming process). When the source has been located, it is subjected to an analysis and storage process occurring in the cortex. Any subsequent reaction (e.g. attack or flight) is based on instinct, past experience or cognitive process. This study investigates under what circumstances an auditory stimulus causes an eye movement. The particular setup, firstly presented by us, attempts to trigger eye movements using a virtual sound source. The experimental results lead to the development of a flow diagram of related information processing in the brain; this may be the beginning of a new method for the diagnosis of central hearing disorders.

Subjects and Method

In 45 volunteers with no eye, neurological or hearing disorders the following laboratory setup was used: the volunteer was placed in a dark, sound-shielded room and subjected to pink noise that is generated using a stereophonic dummy-head according to the principles established by Platte and Laws [4]. The resulting stimulus, presented via headphones from a tape recorder appears as a localized source of sound to the listener. This noise was recorded via a precision impulse sound level meter on channel 1 of an

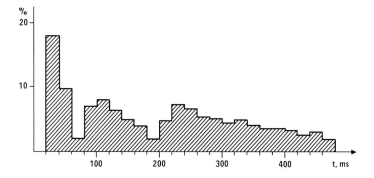

Fig. 1. Distribution of delay in percent (independent of angle).

ENG recorder. The corresponding eye movements of the volunteer were simultaneously recorded on channel 2 of the same recorder.

A random pattern was used to vary the perceived horizontal location of the source of sound. The angle used to describe the source location corresponded to that angle through which the head must turn to face the source directly. The sensors were connected in such a manner that eye movements to the right were recorded on the graph as an upward deflection. The volunteer was instructed to concentrate on the noise from the headphones, no other direction was given. After zeroing and final check of the setup the noise was offered with a maximum noise level of 60 dB(A). The ENG recorder was operating at 25 mm/s corresponding to 40 ms per 1 mm movement of the paper.

Analysis of the measurements included the following: (1) delay between stimulation and response; (2) frequency of reaction; (3) relation between satisfactory response and angle of perceived source; (4) relation between satisfactory response and delay.

In this context 'satisfactory response' is defined as responding to a perceived right-hand source with saccadic eye movements to the right, specifically if triple repetition of the stimulus caused at least two glances in that direction within 1 s.

Results

1,440 stimuli were administered, corresponding to 48 tests for each volunteer. In 23 instances (1.6%) no reaction was observed. Of the remaining 1,417 tests, 306 (21%) responded with one eye movement; 497 (35%) responded with two eye movements, and 614 (43%) responded with three eye movements. Figure 1 shows graphically the distribution of response delays. Three pronounced peaks are evident, the first between 20 and 60 ms, the second between 80 and 160 ms and the third between 240 and 340 ms. The graph also illustrates that immediate eye movements occur more often and exhibit less deviation compared to delayed responses. Statistic evaluation of the measurements has also revealed that stimuli located on the right produced more consistent results, i.e. the reactions could be observed more often.

Discussion

Research of anatomy and physiology by other authors, notably of auditory transmission by Harrison and Howe [1], and the investigation of eye movements by Leigh and Zee [3], have established a connection between the medial superior olive nucleus and the paramedian, parapontine nuclei of the formatio reticularis, the so-called saccadic center. Similarly, there is evidence of transmission between the lemniscus lateralis and the brachium colliculi inferioris, as well as between the cortex, the colliculus inferior region and the saccadic center itself.

According to the literature a reflex is defined as: 'involuntary muscle contractions triggered by a central processor which is subjected to external stimuli'. In this particular experimental setup saccadic eye movements are triggered by auditory stimuli without intervention or processing by higher, more cognitive levels of the brain. Vossius' [6] calculations show that the delay between stimulation of the saccadic center and the corresponding eye movements is of the order of 5–10 ms. Research by Klöss and Fischer [2] on early evoked potentials supports 10 ms as the accepted standard delay to transmit an auditory stimulus to the brain stem region. Adding the two means that at least a 20-ms delay is needed to trigger eye movements. Previous research supports the following typical delays in the transmission of auditory stimuli: 5–10 ms to reach the medial nucleus of the superior olive, 9–13 ms to reach the colliculus inferior.

Response delays to auditory stimuli of the order of 10–24 ms indicate processing by the corpus geniculatum mediale, longer delays are associated with processing by the cortex. An eye movement triggered by the brain at the level of the superior olive complex in response to an auditory stimulus typically occurs with a delay of 20–40 ms. A delay of 23–80 ms (and above) suggests that processing of the stimulus was handled by the colliculus inferior, while 34–200 ms indicates the reaction originated in parts of the cortex. The results of the experiment meet the above guidelines. Based on the findings we conclude that eye movements are an involuntary reaction or reflex only if the associated delay is in the 20- to 40-ms range.

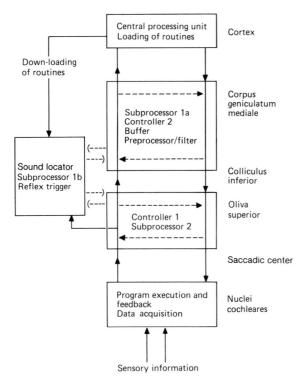

Fig. 2. Cybernetic model of the control of eye movement in response to directional hearing.

The flow diagram in figure 2 graphically illustrates the correlation between a localized source of sound and the scanning of the eyes in the same direction. The central processing unit ZNS loads routines based on information which after some filtering and preprocessing was received via subordinated control units (corpus geniculatum mediale and superior olive). In our case the routine selected is 'visual scanning for source of sound'. The information to be processed has also been assigned a ranking based on a psycho-physical assessment. Based on the processing done by the central processing unit the priority of the associated task (vigilance) in the subordinated processors may be increased or decreased. The effect of this alertness and the aforementioned ranking of the signal may add or cancel each other. If the vigilance is very high (state of alarm), then a reaction to the stimulus may be dispatched at the level of the superior olive (alternate control center). This was established by Shimazu [5] who demonstrated inhibitory and excitatory neuron networks that influence the saccadic center.

The ZNS may be able under certain circumstances to transmit a reflex action directly to the superior olive complex (without involving the corpus geniculatum mediale) via the corticocochlear tract with the colliculus inferior acting as subordinate processor. In this mode the colliculus inferior probably acts as encoder for the sound direction and also handles the reflex response. This path would significantly shorten the processing delay with a correspondingly faster response. If processing is done at the normal state of alertness, then control typically rests with the c. geniculatum mediale (labelled 1a) which has a buffer function, permitting it to pass the stimulus information on to higher levels if required. For this work a tight link to the colliculus inferior (labelled 1b) exists.

This flow diagram is an attempt to model the reflex responses exhibited by saccadic eye movements in response to directional sound. The reader should keep in mind that a delayed, cognitive response (long delay) would not limit subordinate processing. Instead the complete response is the summation of reactions triggered by all processors.

References

1   Harrison, J.M.; Howe, M.E.: Anatomy of the afferent auditory nervous system of mammals. Anatomy of the descending auditory system; in Keidel, Neff, Handbook of sensory physiology, vol. V/1, chap. 9–11 (Springer, Berlin 1974).
2   Klös, G.; Fischer, P.A.: Frühe akustisch evozierte Potentiale in der neurologischen Diagnostik. Diagnostik *17:* Nr. 13 (1984).
3   Leigh, R.J.; Zee, D.S.: The neurology of eye movement. Contemporary Neurol. Ser. (Davis, Philadelphia 1985).
4   Platte, H.J.; Laws, P.: Die Vorne-Ortung bei der kopfbezogenen Stereofonie. Radio Mentor Elektronic *3:* 97–100 (1976).
5   Shimazu, H.: Neuronal organisation of the premotor system controlling horizontal conjugate eye movements and vestibular nystagmus. Adv. Neurol. *39:* 565–588 (1983).
6   Vossius, G.: Das System der Augenbewegungen. I.Z. Biol. *112:* 27–57 (1960).

Dethard Nagel, MD, ENT-Department, University Clinic of Ulm,
Prittwitzstrasse 43, D-7900 Ulm (FRG)

Adv. Oto-Rhino-Laryng., vol. 41, pp. 127–133 (Karger, Basel 1988)

Response Characteristics of Different Size Vestibulospinal Neurons to Roll Tilt of the Animal and Neck Rotation in Decerebrate Cats with the Cerebellum Intact[1]

O. Pompeiano, D. Manzoni, A.R. Marchand, G. Stampacchia

Dipartimento di Fisiologia e Biochimica, Università di Pisa, Pisa, Italy

Introduction

In decerebrate cats submitted to bilateral ablation of the medial cortico-nuclear zone of the cerebellum, Boyle and Pompeiano [3] have recorded the activity of lateral vestibular nucleus (LVN) neurons antidromically identified as projecting to the lumbosacral segments of the cord (lVS neurons), and studied the relation between their resting discharge or response characteristics to excitatory labyrinth and neck afferent volleys and the cell size inferred from the conduction velocity of the corresponding vestibulospinal axon. They tried in this way to find out whether the spontaneous discharge as well as the induced response of these neurons were determined by neuronal properties related to cell size [9, 11], or whether they depended mainly upon synaptic organization, so that a differential control of particular neuronal groups by the relevant input systems could result [4, 11].

Since the paleocerebellum exerts a direct inhibitory influence on LVN neurons [1, 2, 8, 10], we decided to record the activity of lVS neurons in decerebrate cats but with the cerebellum intact. By comparing the resting discharge as well as the response characteristics of different size lVS neurons to labyrinth and neck stimulations, as recorded in these preparations with those previously obtained in partially cerebellectomized cats [3], we could obtain information about the role that the inhibitory area of the cerebellum

[1] This study was supported by the NIH Grant NS 07685-19 and a grant from the Ministero Pubblica Istruzione, Roma, Italy.

exerts on the static and dynamic properties of different size LVN neurons projecting to the lumbosacral segments of the spinal cord.

Methods

The experiments were performed in precollicular decerebrate cats with the cerebellum intact, paralysed with pancuronium bromide (Pavulon, Organon, Oss, The Netherlands, 0.6 mg/kg/h, i.v.) and artificially ventilated. The animal's head was placed in a stereotaxic frame and pitched 10° nose-down. The activity of 129 LVN neurons antidromically activated by electrical stimulation of the spinal cord between T_{12} and L_1 was recorded in the animal at rest and tested during rotation about the longitudinal axis either of the animal (labyrinth input) or of the neck (cervical input) at the standard parameters of 0.026 Hz, ±10° [6, 7]. The unit activity was processed on-line with a computer system equipped with a fast Fourier analyzer. A spectral analysis of the angular input (animal or neck rotation) and of the output (unit activity) was performed and the gain (imp./s/°) and phase angle of the first harmonic of response were evaluated, the latter being the difference in arc degrees between the peak of the fundamental component of response and the peak of the side-down animal or neck displacement.

Results

In the present experiments, as well as in previous experiments performed after ablation of the paleocerebellum [3], the lVS units responsive and unresponsive to animal tilt or neck rotation were particularly located within the dorsocaudal part of LVN and covered the entire range of conduction velocity. The resting discharge of the spontaneously firing lVS neurons tested during vestibular stimulation (24.5 ± 15.7 SD imp./s; n = 108) was significantly lower than that obtained after partial cerebellectomy (44.1 ± 23.8 SD imp./s, n = 136) [3]. Moreover, the units responsive to vestibular stimulation displayed a lower resting discharge rate (21.3 ± 15.4 SD imp./s) than the unresponsive ones (29.9 ± 14.7 SD imp./s) (t-test, p <0.01), a finding which did not occur when the paleocerebellum was removed. Similar results were also found for the population of 95 spontaneously firing lVS neurons tested to neck rotation.

In addition to the findings reported above, a *slight* negative correlation was found between the resting discharge of the whole population of lVS neurons responsive and unresponsive to animal tilt and neck rotation and the conduction velocity of the corresponding axons, so that the faster the conduction velocity the lower was the unit discharge rate at rest (paired rank,

Erratum

Please note that in table I on p. 130 some digits have erroneously been lost. This is the new, corrected table I of the paper "Response Characteristics of Different Size Vestibulospinal Neurons to Roll Tilt of the Animal and Neck Rotation in Decerebrate Cats with the Cerebellum Intact" by O. Pompeiano et al.

Table I. Effects of sinusoidal stimulation of labyrinth and neck receptors (at 0.026 Hz, $\pm 10°$) on the activity of slow and fast neurons

	Number of responsive (R) units	Resting discharge rate of R-units	Gain of R-units	Phase angle of R-units			Number of unresponsive units	Resting discharge rate of unresponsive units
				side-down	side-up	intermediate		
Labyrinth input								
$\leq$90m/s	26	22.9±16.4 n=24 *	0.41±0.39 *	+31.4±25.4 n=16	+175.4±37.2 n=5	n=5	24	35.8±13.3 n=23 **
>90/ms	50	20.4±15.0 n=44	0.51±0.46	+22.1±22.9 n=35	−166.6±32.4 n=10	n=5	18	22.0±13.0 n=17
Neck input								
$\leq$90m/s	31	28.6±17.3 n=29 **	0.45±0.43 *	+56.5±30.7 n=4	−130.2±19.4 n=25	n=2	15	29.0±16.2 *
>90m/s	44	17.2±14.4 n=41	0.51±0.39	+55.4±8.9 n=4	−127.2±17.2 n=34	n=6	10	26.0±10.6

Resting discharge rate, in imp./s; gain of the first harmonic, in imp./s/°; phase angle of the first harmonic, in degrees of phase lead (positive values) or phase lag (negative values) with respect to the side-down animal or neck displacement. For each of these parameters, the mean ±SD is given. Notice that 11 units unresponsive to labyrinth stimulation (1 slow and 10 fast) and 9 units unresponsive to neck stimulation (2 slow and 7 fast) were disregarded because they were silent at rest. *No significant difference (t-test); **$p < 0.01$ (t-test).

p <0.01). This correlation, however, affected the units unresponsive but not those responsive to vestibular stimulation; the opposite occurred for the units tested to neck stimulation (table I). These findings differ from those obtained after partial cerebellectomy [3], where a *prominent* negative correlation was found between resting discharge and conduction velocity, i.e. cell size of all the lVS units irrespective of their responsiveness to labyrinth or neck input (paired rank, p <0.001).

The proportion of lVS neurons responsive to standard parameters of animal (76 out of 129 lVS units, i.e. 58.9%) and neck rotation (75 out of 109 lVS units, i.e. 68.8%) in the present experiments, as well as their response gains (0.47 ± 0.44 SD imp./s/° for the labyrinth responses and 0.49 ± 0.40 SD imp./s/° for the neck responses) closely corresponded to the values obtained after removal of the paleocerebellum [3]. As to the response patterns, most of the lVS neurons recorded in the present experiments were excited during side-down animal tilt (51 out of 76 units, i.e. 67.1%) and side-up neck rotation (59 out of 75 units, i.e. 78.6%), while after cerebellectomy the proportion of lVS neurons showing these response patterns (26.3 and 46.2%, respectively) decreased in favour of units which displayed the opposite ones [3]. All these findings indicate that at least in decerebrate animals the cerebellum is not very effective in modifying the average responsiveness and gains of the lVS neurons to animal tilt and neck rotation, but rather intervenes in determining their response patterns.

It is of interest that in the present experiments the two populations of lVS units showing the reciprocal patterns of response to animal tilt or neck rotation were not distinguishable insofar as they covered the whole range of resting discharge and the whole spectrum of conduction velocity of the corresponding axons; however, the average gains of the units showing the predominant response patterns (excitation during side-down animal tilt or side-up neck rotation) were significantly higher than those displayed by the remaining populations of units (t-test, p <0.01 and p <0.05 for gain differences of labyrinth and neck responses, respectively). These differences in gain, however, were not observed after cerebellectomy [3].

Finally, if we consider the response gains of the lVS neurons to standard parameters of animal tilt and neck rotation independently from their response patterns, it appeared that the values obtained in the present experiments were on the average slightly, although not significantly, higher for the large size neurons (conduction velocity of axons >90 m/s) than for the small size neurons (conduction velocity of axons ⩽90 m/s) (table I). Similar results had previously been obtained in cerebellectomized cats [3].

Discussion

The demonstration that the resting discharge of the lVS neurons recorded in the present experiments was lower than that obtained in partially cerebellectomized cats [3] indicates that the cerebellar vermis exerts a tonic inhibitory influence on lVS neurons. Indeed, most of the units were located in the dcLVN, which represents the main area of termination of the cerebellar corticovestibular projection [5], thus receiving the inhibitory influence of the corresponding Purkinje cells [1, 2, 8, 10]. This influence was particularly prominent on the lVS units responsive to animal tilt and neck rotation as shown by their lower resting discharge with respect to the unresponsive units.

It is of interest that in the present experiments the negative correlation between resting discharge rate and conduction velocity, i.e. cell size of all the lVS neurons responsive and unresponsive to animal tilt and neck rotation was much smaller than that obtained after partial cerebellectomy [3].

If we assume that the excitatory (labyrinthine and extralabyrinthine) afferents impinging on the LVN neurons are homogeneously distributed, thus making an equal number of synaptic contacts with different size lVS neurons, then the prominent negative correlation between resting discharge and conduction velocity of the lVS units recorded in cerebellectomized animals could be in agreement with the 'size principle' which states that the smaller the size of the neurons, the more effective is the corresponding input in exciting them due to their higher input resistance [9, 11]. The reduced slope of the regression line relating the resting discharge of the lVS neurons to the conduction velocity of the corresponding axon in the present experiments with the cerebellum intact depends on the fact that the small size lVS neurons, particularly those responsive to vestibular stimulation, fired at a lower rate with respect to cerebellectomized preparations, while the resting discharge of the large size lVS neurons was not much affected by the cerebellar ablation. These findings can be attributed to a more prominent tonic inhibitory influence of the cerebellum on the small size with respect to the large size neurons.

The greater susceptibility of the small size lVS neurons to corticocerebellar inhibition can in part at least be attributed to their higher input resistance. They might also receive from the cerebellar Purkinje cells a higher number of inhibitory synaptic contacts on the cell body and/or proximal dendrites, which counteract the excess of input excitation.

The demonstration that in preparations with the cerebellum intact, a proportion of lVS neurons did not respond to animal tilt and neck rotation excludes that the lVS neurons represent a homogeneous population differing only in cell size. Moreover, the observation that the two populations of responsive and unresponsive units covered the entire range of conduction velocity indicates that there are differences in connectivity of the same afferents impinging on lVS neurons of comparable size. Similar results were also obtained after cerebellectomy [3].

Obviously we cannot exclude that the behaviour of the lVS neurons responsive to labyrinth and neck stimulations is specified by intrinsic neuronal properties related to the cell size [9, 11]. Strict application of this hypothesis, however, is not supported by the experimental findings. First of all it appears that in the present experiments the response gains of the lVS units displaying the predominant response patterns to vestibular and neck stimulations (i.e. excitation during side-down animal tilt and side-up neck rotation) were on the average significantly higher than those of the units showing the other response patterns; yet, no differences were found in the average conduction velocity and thus in the cell size of these populations of units. These differences in gains, which were not observed after cerebellec-tomy [3], suggest that in the intact preparations afferent pathways originating from populations of otolith and neck receptors having opposite polarization vectors are not homogeneously distributed among the different size lVS neurons. Furthermore, the gain of all the unit responses to standard param-eters of animal tilt and neck rotation tended to be higher for the large than for the small neurons. Similar results were also obtained in individual experiments after cerebellectomy.

This finding suggests that the influence of size on input resistance is cancelled and possibly overwhelmed by the influence of size on the number of synaptic contacts [12] made by the afferent pathways driven during dynamic stimulation of labyrinth and neck receptors. The possibility that inhibitory synaptic contacts of cerebellar origin also contribute to increase the response gain of these large size neurons cannot be excluded, since during vestibular or neck stimulation Purkinje cells of the cerebellar vermis usually discharge 180° out of phase with respect to the lVS neurons [6, 7].

References

1   Akaike, T.: Electrophysiological analysis of cerebellar corticovestibular and fastigio-vestibular projections to the lateral vestibular nucleus in the cat. Brain Res. *272:* 223–235 (1983).

2   Akaike, T.; Fanardjian, V.V.; Ito, M.; Nakajima, H.: Cerebellar control of the vestibulospinal tract cells in rabbit. Exp. Brain Res. *18:* 446–463 (1973).
3   Boyle, R.; Pompeiano, O.: Relation between cell size and response characteristics of vestibulospinal neurons to labyrinth and neck inputs. J. Neurosci. *1:* 1052–1065 (1981).
4   Burke, R.E.: The role of synaptic organization in the control of motor unit activity during movement; in Granit, Pompeiano, Progress in brain research, vol. 50, pp. 61–67 (Elsevier, Amsterdam 1979).
5   Corvaja, N.; Pompeiano, O.: Identification of cerebellar corticovestibular neurons retrogradely labeled with horseradish peroxidase. Neuroscience *4:* 507–515 (1979).
6   Denoth, F.; Magherini, P.C.; Pompeiano, O.; Stanojević, M.: Responses of Purkinje cells of the cerebellar vermis to neck and macular inputs. Pflügers Arch. *381:* 87–98 (1979).
7   Denoth, F.; Magherini, P.C.; Pompeiano, O.; Stanojević, M.: Responses of Purkinje cells of cerebellar vermis to sinusoidal rotation of neck. J. Neurophysiol. *43:* 46–59 (1980).
8   Fanardjian, V.V.; Sarkissian, V.A.: Spatial organization of the cerebellar corticovestibular projection in the cat. Neuroscience *5:* 551–558 (1980).
9   Henneman, E.; Mendell, L.M.: Functional organization of motoneuron pool and its inputs; in Brooks, Handbook of physiology, vol. II, pp. 423–507 (Am. Physiological Society, Bethesda 1981).
10 Ito, M.: Cerebellar control of the vestibular neurons: physiology and pharmacology; in Brodal, Pompeiano, Progress in brain research, vol. 37, pp. 377–390 (Elsevier, Amsterdam 1972).
11 Stuart, D.G.; Enoka, R.M.: Motoneurons, motor units, and the size principle; in Rosenberg, The clinical neurosciences, sect. 5, pp. 471–517 (Churchill-Livingstone, New York 1983).
12 Zucker, R.S.: Theoretical implications of the size principle of motoneuron recruitment. J. theor. Biol. *38:* 587–596 (1973).

Prof. O. Pompeiano, Dipartimento di Fisiologia e Biochimica, Università di Pisa, Via S. Zeno 31, I-56100 Pisa (Italy)

Adv. Oto-Rhino-Laryng., vol. 41, pp. 134–141 (Karger, Basel 1988)

Gain Regulation of the Vestibulospinal Reflex following Microinjection of a ß-Adrenergic Agonist or Antagonist into the Locus Coeruleus and the Dorsal Pontine Reticular Formation[1]

G. Stampacchia, P. D'Ascanio, E. Horn, O. Pompeiano

Dipartimento di Fisiologia e Biochimica, Università di Pisa, Pisa, Italy

Introduction

The present knowledge about the control of posture and the gain regulation of the vestibulospinal (VS) reflex in mammals is mainly based on investigations performed in decerebrate cats in which the EMG activity of forelimb extensor muscles was recorded in the animal at rest as well as during sinusoidal stimulation of macular labyrinth receptors [1, 8, 14, 17]. These experiments have led to a minimal model, which includes not only excitatory VS neurons originating from the lateral vestibular nucleus (LVN) and acting on ipsilateral extensor motoneurons [12], but also inhibitory reticulospinal neurons originating from the medial aspect of the medullary reticular formation [9]. It appears, in particular, that the increased contraction of limb extensor muscles which occurs during side-down roll tilt of the animal [6, 10, 16] depends on both an increased discharge of excitatory VS neurons and a reduced discharge of medullary inhibitory reticulospinal (mRS) neurons [13].

There is now evidence that the inhibitory mRS neurons, which fire at a very low rate in the animals at rest, are tonically excited by cholinergic and self-excitatory cholinoceptive neurons located in the dorsal pontine reticular formation (pRF). On the other hand, the activity of this pontine area is under the tonic inhibitory control of norepinephrine (NE)-containing locus coeruleus (LC) neurons, which are also self-inhibitory and send afferent projections to the underlying reticular neurons [5]. An increased discharge of the

[1] This study was supported by the NIH Grant NS 07685–19 and a grant from the Ministero Pubblica Istruzione, Roma, Italy.

cholinergic pRF neurons and the related inhibitory mRS neurons which occurs either following unilateral injection into the dorsal pRF region of minute amounts of cholinomimetic substances, like carbachol or bethanechol [1, 17], or after local injection into the LC of one side of the α_2-adrenergic agonist clonidine which suppresses the activity of the corresponding neurons [8, 14], while reducing the postural activity in limb extensors, greatly increased the gain of the EMG responses of the ipsilateral triceps brachii to sinusoidal labyrinth stimulation.

The following experiments were performed to find out whether ß-adrenoceptors located on dorsal pRF neurons and/or LC neurons are involved in the noradrenergic-mediated control of posture and vestibulospinal reflexes.

Methods

Experiments were performed in precollicular decerebrate cats with good symmetric extensor rigidity of both forelimbs. The multiunit EMG activity of the medial head of the triceps brachii was bilaterally recorded in the animal at rest as well as during roll tilt of the animal at the frequency of 0.15 Hz, $\pm 10°$, following the method described in a previous study [10]. Sequential pulse density histograms were obtained by averaging data of 6 sweeps. These stimulation sequences were usually repeated at regular intervals of about 5–10 min for several hours, before and after injection of minute doses of a ß-adrenergic agonist or antagonist into the LC or in the surrounding pontine reticular structures. The digital data related to the averaged EMG responses were processed on-line with a computer system (PET, 2001-8C) which performed the Fourier and correlation analysis as well as the transfer function of the system. Mean firing rate of the multiunit EMG activity (base frequency: imp./s), gain (imp./s/°) and phase angle (degrees) of the first harmonic of the output with respect to the peak of the side-down displacement of the animal ipsilateral to the side of recording were evaluated.

For the injections of drugs, a vertically oriented stainless steel cannula, with a diameter at the tip of 0.5 mm, was lowered stereotaxically in different dorsal pontine structures. Propranolol (ß-antagonist) or isoproterenol (ß-agonist), which act on both β_1- and β_2-adrenoceptors, were injected locally into the pRF (at the stereotaxic coordinates of P2.5, L2.5/3.5, II-3.5/4.5) or into the LC (at P2.5. L2.5/2.8, H-2.0/2.5), respectively. The drugs were dissolved in sterile saline (0.9% NaCl) stained with the dye pontamine (5%) as a marker for the injection site. Usually 0.25 µl of a solution of propranolol or isoproterenol at the concentration of 4.5–9 µg/µl of sterile saline (i.e.. 1.1–2.2 µg) were injected on one side. Drug delivery was performed following the methods described in a previous paper [1]. In some control experiments the cats received a local injection of 0.25 µl of the solvent.

At the end of each experiment the brain was removed and fixed in 10% formaline. It was then possible to identify the precise site of the tip of the cannula, as well as the extent of the nerve tissue stained with the blue dye on serial frozen sections of the brain stem stained with neutral red.

Results

After decerebration, the animals showed a good rigidity in the four limbs and a symmetric EMG activity on forelimb extensors of both sides. In all the experiments a sinusoidal modulation of the multiunit EMG activity of the medial head of the triceps brachii was obtained during roll tilt of the animal at the standard parameters of 0.15 Hz, $\pm 10°$, which was characterized by an increased activity during side-down and a decreased activity during side-up tilt of the animal (α-responses). Moreover, the peak of the responses was closely related to the extreme animal displacement, thus being attributed to stimulation of position-sensitive macular (utricular) receptors.

Microinjection of the β-antagonist propranolol into the dorsal aspect of the pRF of one side produced a postural asymmetry, characterized by a prominent decrease of the extensor tonus in the ipsilateral limbs, while the decerebrate rigidity was not greatly modified in the contralateral limbs. After injection, the gain of the multiunit EMG response of the triceps brachii to animal tilt increased on the ipsilateral side, but slightly decreased on the contralateral side (fig. 1a). These findings were still obtained even when the base frequency was kept constant by increasing or decreasing the static stretch of the muscle, thus leading to an averaged muscular activity comparable to that obtained prior to the injection. The response pattern usually remained unchanged on both sides (α-responses). In some instances, however, it reversed on the contralateral side, as shown by an increased EMG activity of the corresponding triceps brachii during side-up and a decreased activity during side-down animal tilt (β-responses).

Fig. 1. Effects of local injections of a β-antagonist into different pontine structures on the response gain of the ipsilateral and the contralateral triceps brachii to roll tilt of the animal at the frequency of 0.15 Hz, $\pm 10°$. Precollicular, decerebrate cats. *a* Experiment 1: The gains of the averaged multiunit responses of the triceps brachii of both sides to animal tilt were evaluated at different time intervals before and after local injection of the β-antagonist propranolol (1.1 µg) into the pRF of the right side (inset, hatched area). *b* Experiment 4: The response gains of the triceps brachii of both sides to animal tilt were evaluated before and after local injections of the β-agonist isoproterenol (1.1 µg) either into the pRF (1) or into the LC (2) of the right side (inset, hatched area). Note that injection 1, outside the LC, was ineffective. Each dot represents the mean value of 6 averaged responses. The arrows indicate the time of injection (0 min.) Ipsi = the injection side; Contra = the opposite side.

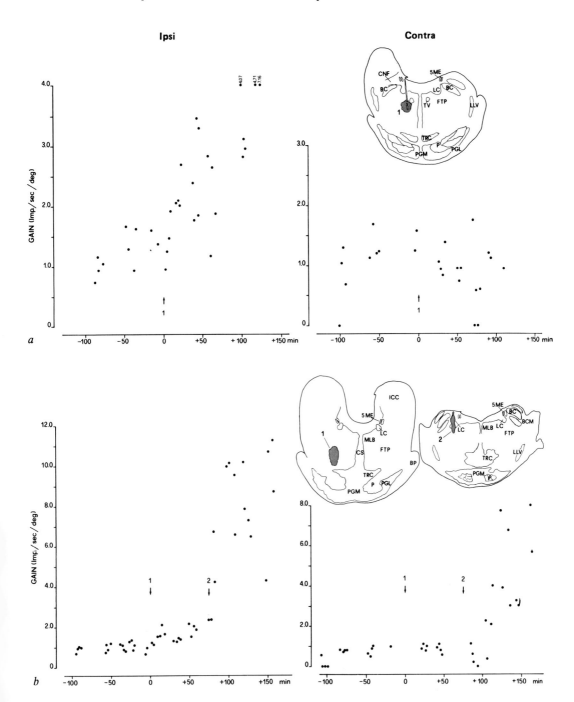

A detailed analysis of the results indicated that in two experiments (exps. 1, 3), the mean gain of the VS reflex of the ipsilateral muscle increased significantly from 0.81 ± 0.48 SD imp./s/° (n=21 groups of averaged responses) before, to 1.82 ± 1.07 SD imp./s/° (n=69) after drug treatment, while the phase angle calculated only for the α-responses shifted from an average lead of $+20.2 \pm 12.3°$ SD (n=17) to $+11.8 \pm 15.3°$ SD (n=68). On the contralateral side, however, the mean gain of the VS reflex decreased significantly from 0.98 ± 0.44 SD imp./s/° (n=20) before, to 0.66 ± 0.34 SD imp./s/° (n=46) after drug injection, while the phase angle calculated only for the α-responses shifted from an average lead of $+4.9 \pm 11.3°$ SD (n=20) to $+1.2 \pm 16.3°$ SD (n=33), respectively.

Local injection of the β-agonist isoproterenol into the LC of one side decreased the spontaneous EMG activity of the ipsilateral triceps brachii and to a lesser extent also that of the contralateral muscle. The same injection also increased the amplitude of modulation and thus the response gain of the forelimb extensors to the same parameters of labyrinth stimulation, both ipsilaterally and to a lesser extent also contralaterally to the side of the injection (fig. 1b, injection 2). However, no change in the α-pattern of responses was observed.

In particular, in two experiments (exps. 4, 5), the mean gain of the VS reflex of the ipsilateral muscle increased significantly from 0.83 ± 0.26 SD imp./s/° (n=33 groups of averaged responses) before, to 6.17 ± 3.61 SD imp./s/° (n=20) after drug treatment, while the phase angle shifted from an average lead of $+12.0 \pm 8.6°$ SD to $+26.7 \pm 13.5°$ SD. As to the contralateral side, the gain of the VS reflex increased on the average from 0.79 ± 0.30 SD imp./s/° (n=20) before, to 3.10 ± 1.87 SD imp./s/° (n=31) after drug injection, while the phase angle of the responses varied from an average lead of $+8.8 \pm 9.4°$ SD (n=20) to $+20.7 \pm 10.4°$ SD (n=25), respectively.

The results described above were site-specific; in fact, an injection performed about 2.0 mm rostroventrally to the LC did not produce any postural and reflex change, indicating that the isoproterenol effect was brought about by β-receptors in the LC (fig, 1b, injection 1). Moreover, the effects could be attributed to activation of β-receptors since propranolol, injected after isoproterenol into the LC, antagonized the effect of the β-agonist, as shown by the reduced gain of responses of the triceps brachii of both sides to labyrinth stimulation. Control experiments indicated that the gain of the VS reflex was not influenced by injecting an equal volume (0.25 μl) of the solvent either into the LC (exp. 18) or into the dorsal pRF (exps. 15, 20).

Discussion

The presence of β-receptors into the brain stem, including pontine reticular structures, was recently demonstrated both in binding studies [11] as well as by using histofluorescent [7] and autoradiographic methods [15]. The main result of the present experiments was that unilateral injection of minute doses of the β-antagonist propranolol into the dorsal aspect of the pRF not only reduced the postural activity in the ipsilateral limb extensors, but also increased the amplitude of modulation and thus the response gain of the corresponding triceps brachii to labyrinth stimulation. Just the opposite effects were obtained contralaterally to the side of the injection.

In order to explain these findings, we postulated that the β-antagonist blocks the inhibitory influence exerted by the NE-containing LC neurons on the ipsilateral dorsal pRF, where cholinergic and self-excitatory cholinoceptive neurons are located [for references, see ref. 5]. The increased discharge of these pRF neurons and the related inhibitory mRS neurons would lead to a decreased postural activity in the ipsilateral limbs. Moreover, for a given labyrinth signal, the higher the firing rate of the mRS neurons in the animal at rest, the greater the disinhibition which affects the ipsilateral extensor motoneurons during side-down tilt. These motoneurons would then respond more efficiently to the same excitatory volleys elicited by given parameters of stimulation, thus leading to an increased gain of the EMG responses of forelimb extensor muscles to labyrinth stimulation.

The inhibitory influence exerted by the LC neurons on the dorsal pRF and the related inhibitory mRS neurons was also depressed in our experiments by local injection into the LC of the β-agonist isoproterenol, which inhibits the spontaneous firing of the noradrenergic LC neurons, as shown by iontophoretic studies [2, 3]. In this instance, inactivation of the NE-containing LC neurons of one side produced by the β-agonist not only decreased the postural activity of the ipsilateral limbs, but also increased the response gain of the triceps brachii of both sides. That the LC of one side keeps under its tonic inhibitory control the cholinergic pRF region not only of the ipsilateral but also, to a lesser extent, of the contralateral side is supported by the results of previous experiments, showing that an increase in the response gain of the contralateral as well as of the ipsilateral triceps brachii to animal tilt was also obtained either after electrolytic lesion of the LC of one side [4] or after inactivation of the LC neurons produced by local injection of the α_2-adrenergic agonist clonidine into the LC [8, 14].

In conclusion, it appears that the NE-containing LC neurons exert a critical role in the control of posture as well as in the gain regulation of the VS reflex. This role involves, in part at least, an inhibitory influence that the LC neurons exert on the pRF neurons and the related mRS system by acting through β-adrenoceptors. There is also evidence that the background discharge of the noradrenergic LC neurons is under the tonic inhibitory control of NE, which may act not only on α_2-adrenoceptors as shown by clonidine injections, but also on β-receptors. Experiments are required to find out the relative influence that the subtypes β-adrenoceptors (i.e. β_1- and B_2-receptors) exert on posture as well as on the gain of the VS reflex.

References

1 Barnes, C.D.; D'Ascanio, P.; Pompeiano, O.; Stampacchia, G.: Effects of microinjection of cholinergic agonists into the pontine reticular formation on the gain of vestibulospinal reflexes in decerebrate cats. Arch. ital. Biol. *125:* 71–105 (1987).

2 Cedarbaum, J.M.; Aghajanian, G.K.: Noradrenergic neurons of the locus coeruleus: inhibition by epinephrine and activation by the α-antagonist piperoxane. Brain Res. *112:* 413–419 (1976).

3 Cedarbaum, J.M.; Aghajanian, G.K.: Catecholamine receptors on locus coeruleus neurons: pharmacological characterization. Eur. J. Pharmacol. *44:* 375–385 (1977).

4 D'Ascanio, P.; Bettini, E.; Pompeiano, O.: Tonic inhibitory influences of locus coeruleus on the response gain of limb extensors to sinusoidal labyrinth and neck stimulations. Arch. ital. Biol. *123:* 69–100 (1985).

5 D'Ascanio, P.; Pompeiano, O.; Stampacchia, G.: Noradrenergic and cholinergic mechanisms responsible for the gain regulation of vestibulospinal reflexes; in Pompeiano, Allum, Progress in brain research, vol. 76, pp. 361–374 (Elsevier, Amsterdam 1988).

6 Ezure, K.; Wilson, V.J.: Interaction of tonic neck and vestibular reflexes in the forelimb of the decerebrate cat. Exp. Brain Res. *54:* 289–292 (1984).

7 Hess, A.: Visualization of beta-adrenergic receptor sites with fluorescent beta-adrenergic blocker probes — or autofluorescent granules? Brain Res. *160:* 533–538 (1979).

8 Horn, E.; D'Ascanio, P.; Pompeiano, O.; Stampacchia, G.: Pontine reticular origin of cholinergic excitatory afferents to the locus coeruleus controlling the gain of vestibulospinal and cervicospinal reflexes in decerebrate cats. Arch. ital. Biol. *125:* 273–304 (1987).

9 Magoun, H.W.; Rhines, R.: Spasticity. The stretch-reflex and extrapyramidal systems, pp. VII–59 (Thomas, Springfield 1947).

10 Manzoni, D.; Pompeiano, O.; Srivastava, U.C.; Stampacchia, G.: Responses of forelimb extensors to sinusoidal stimulation of macular labyrinth and neck receptors. Arch. ital. Biol. *121:* 205–214 (1983).

11 Pompeiano, M.: Distribuzione e parziale caratterizzazione dei recettori β-adrenergici nelle aree inibitorie del cervello di gatto; MD thesis, Pisa, p. 59 (1986).

12 Pompeiano, O.: Vestibulo-spinal relationships; in Naunton, The vestibular system, pp. 147–180 (Academic Press, New York 1975).

13 Pompeiano, O..: A comparison of the response characteristics of vestibulospinal and reticulospinal neurons to labyrinth and neck inputs; in Barnes, Research topics in physiology, vol. 6, pp. 87–140 (Academic Press, New York 1984).

14 Pompeiano, O.; D'Ascanio, P.; Horn, E.; Stampacchia, G.: Effects of local injection of the α_2-adrenergic agonist clonidine into the locus coeruleus complex on the gain of vestibulospinal and cervicospinal reflexes in decerebrate cats. Arch. ital. Biol. *125:* 225–269 (1987).

15 Rainbow, T.C.; Parsons, B.; Wolfe, B.B.: Quantitative autoradiography of β_1- and β_2-adrenergic receptors in rat brain. Proc. natn. Acad. Sci. USA *81:* 1585–1589 (1984).

16 Schor, R.H.; Miller, A.D.: Vestibular reflexes in neck and forelimb muscles evoked by roll tilt. J. Neurophysiol. *46:* 167–178 (1981).

17 Stampacchia, G.; Barnes, C.D.; D'Ascanio, P.; Pompeiano, O.: Effects of microinjection of a cholinergic agonist into the locus coeruleus on the gain of vestibulospinal reflexes in decerebrate cats. Arch. ital. Biol. *125:* 107–138 (1987).

Prof. O. Pompeiano, Dipartimento di Fisiologia e Biochimica, Università di Pisa, Via S. Zeno 31, I-56100 Pisa (Italy)

Adv. Oto-Rhino-Laryng., vol. 41, pp. 142–145 (Karger, Basel 1988)

Mammalian Macular Organization: A Model Information Network[1]

Muriel D. Ross

NASA Ames Research Center, Moffett Field, Calif., USA

Introduction

Recent ultrastructural findings in rat maculas have demonstrated that type II hair cells are integrated into the neural circuitry innervating type I cells [1, 2]. This work also showed that three kinds of afferent terminal patterns occur. These are U-, M/U- and M-types, illustrated diagrammatically in figure 1. These and other observations were interpreted to indicate that complex processing of information takes place in the mammalian macula. More recent study of a long series of sections through rat utricular macula supports the notion that type II hair cells link calyces and distribute information. This means that maculas are neural networks morphologically organized for parallel processing of linear acceleratory signals. This paper focuses on macular neural connectivity, especially on networks in pars externa encompassing the three different kinds of nerve/terminal patterns. The evident weighting in directional flow of information and possible physiological implications of the findings are discussed.

Material and Methods

Results reported here are based upon study of every fifth section taken from a series of 570 sections through a rat utricular macula. Tissues were prepared similarly to other series [1] in which the primary fixative included 1% osmium tetroxide. Sections were

[1] This research was sponsored by NASA-G-NAG 2-33; NASA-G-NAG 2-325; and NASA-C-NAS-10535.

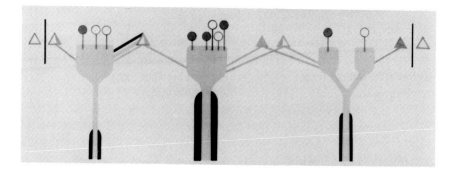

Fig. 1. This diagram is a model of linked terminals which illustrates a weighted, macular information network. It is based upon actual reconstructions, but the weightings are symbolic. The three nerves ending in calyces represent U- (far left), M- (middle) and M/U- (far right) types of nerve patterns. Circles represent type I cells. Triangles are type II cells. The calyx at left has two collaterals, shown as heavy lines. The darker heavy line is an efferent-type; the lighter one is afferent in type. The remaining lines between type II cells and calyces represent synapses. Solid circles and triangles represent a weighting of two, while open circles have a weight of one. Triangles half-filled have a weighting of two in the direction filled. The circuit is stopped at straight lines (left and right), where type II cells cluster.

photographed in a Philips 400 transmission microscope, and the micrographs were assembled as montages. Terminal fields were traced onto acetate from the montages, for further study in 3 dimensions and for reconstruction in network format.

Results

Neural connectivity differs according to location in the macula. In pars externa, all three kinds of terminal are commonly interlinked in weighted fashion (figure 1). By weighting it is meant that there may be one, two or three type II cells forming linkages between the same two calyces. Additionally, synapses between a type II hair cell and a calyx may be weighted because the number of junctions is variable, with from one to three synapses being the most common. The model shown in figure 1 illustrates many of these features.

In contrast, preliminary study of outlying networks in pars externa indicates that they consist only of unmyelinated nerves and their terminals. The networks are far more complex than those at the striola. The nerves intertwine with one another and the calyces often are contiguous. Numerous collaterals, often efferent in type, are evident between calyces and type II cells of the region.

Discussion

Figure 1 is an initial attempt to model a small part of the circuitry observed in pars externa. The model illustrates (1) that maculas process information in parallel; (2) that information flow is not symmetrical but is weighted, and (3) that type II hair cells sometimes distribute information to calyces of all three kinds of nerve terminal patterns. The findings provide a morphological basis for considering the maculas to be weighted information (or neural) networks.

The results mean firstly that a particular nerve response is not related simply to the morphology of its own terminal field, but is also influenced by activity in its neighbors in the network, through shared type II cells. Secondly, a nerve response indicating that the terminal is behaving as though its hair cells have preferred directional orientations [3] may not reflect a resultant of vectors summed by the hair cells. The relationship may be nonlinear, because of weighting in the circuit. Thirdly, regularity or irregularity of discharge patterns may be related, at least in part, to the fact that unmyelinated nerves and their calyces come into close physical contiguity in some areas, increasing the likelihood of electrical interaction between them. This would likely act to synchronize their discharges and make them more regular. In other areas, in contrast, individual nerves stay physically apart from one another and many of the nerves have short or no unmyelinated segments. This leaves the M/U- and M-types, at least, free of the influence of electrical activity in other nearby nerves. U-types linked into these circuits have not yet been followed far enough to determine whether they are also free of the intertwining characteristic of U-types in pars externa. Asynchrony in response to the same, shared information would characterize a mixed network like the one described here. Timing is a method of transmitting information, perhaps (in this case) to signal the direction and speed of acceleration.

Further physiological research is required to increase our understanding of maculas as parallel processors. Nevertheless, the morphology of the networks described here could explain the physiological properties of irregularly and regularly discharging nerves described previously by Goldberg et al. [4] which they, however, largely ascribed to variations in postsynaptic recovery functions.

References

1 Ross, M.D.: Anatomic evidence for peripheral neural processing in mammalian graviceptors. Aviat. Space environ. Med. *56:* 338–343 (1985).
2 Ross, M.D.; Rogers, C.M.; Donovan, K.M.: Innervation patterns in rat saccular macula. Acta oto-lar. *102:* 75–86 (1986).
3 Loe, P.R.; Tomko, D.L.; Werner, G.: The neural signal of angular head position in primary afferent vestibular nerve axons. J. Physiol. *230:* 29–50 (1973).
4 Goldberg, J.M.; Baird, R.A.; Fernandez, C.: Morphophysiological studies of the mammalian vestibular labyrinth; in Correia and Perachio, Contemporary sensory neurobiology, pp. 231–245 (Liss, New York 1985).

Muriel D. Ross, PhD, Chief, Space Biology Branch, NASA Ames Research Center, Moffett Field, CA 94035 (USA)

Adv. Oto-Rhino-Laryng., vol. 41, pp. 146–151 (Karger, Basel 1988)

Postural Control in the Oldest Olds

Ilmari Pyykkö[a], Pirkko Jäntti[b], Heikki Aalto[c]

[a]Department of Otolaryngology, University Hospital of Helsinki,
[b]Geriatric Clinic, Tampere City Hospital, University of Tampere,
[c]Institute of Occupational Health, Helsinki, Finland

Introduction

Accidental falls are commonly encountered by elderly subjects. The mechanism and cause leading to falls has been extensively studied but no common denominator has yet been found that could be used to prevent the falls [Overstall et al., 1977; Barlett et al., 1986; Bauer, 1970]. The purpose of the present study was to evaluate the postural control mechanism in the oldest olds.

Subjects and Methods

Thirteen females and 4 males aged 80–85 years were studied in the Geriatric Research Unit in the City Hospital of Tampere. All subjects were outpatients living on their own. The general health of the subject was surveyed, the vibration sense was tested with a tuning fork from the extremities and an evaluation of tendon reflexes was made.

The force platform was constructed with the strain gauge principle [Aalto et al., 1988]. The force distribution on the platform surface was measured and the centerpoint of force coordinates in fore-aft and lateral directions were recorded during the test and stored in an FM tape recorder for a later analysis.

The postural perturbation was induced by stimulating calf muscles of each leg with vibration, delivered in pseudorandom fashion at different frequencies (fig. 1). The stimulator unit was controlled with a microcomputer and the intensity of vibration was delivered with rotary types of shakers giving a 0.4-mm peak-to-peak amplitude at all frequencies. The duration of posturography measurement was 180 s. A detailed description of the posturographic stimulation is provided elsewhere [Pyykkö et al., 1986b].

For the analysis of the data the posturography signal was fed into a microcomputer. The data were sampled at a frequency of 33.3 Hz. To eliminate artefacts the data were filtered with a 3-point median filter and smoothed with a linear filter (-3 dB point at 3.3

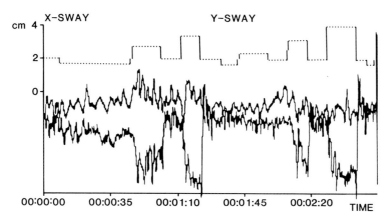

Fig. 1. Computer display of posturography signal. Uppermost tracing = stimulus; middle tracing = fore-aft sway; lowest tracing = lateral sway.

Hz) to remove random noise. The program calculated, among other parameters, sway velocity during stimulation-free and different stimulation conditions. A detailed description of the filtering procedure [Aalto et al., 1988] and data calculation [Pyykkö et al., 1986b] have been provided elsewhere.

The test was conducted in four conditions: (1) on a rigid surface with visual control; (2) on a rigid surface without visual control; (3) on a foam rubber covered surface with visual control, and (4) on a foam rubber covered surface without visual control. The duration of total posturographic testing was 1 h.

The results from the elderly subjects were compared with posturography recordings made in 100 subjects aged 45–55 years collected in a cohort study from different parts of Finland. In the statistical calculation analysis of variance was used. When $p < 0.05$ the statement was considered to be statistically significant.

Results

Rigid Surface with Visual Control

In the oldest olds, when standing with eyes open on a rigid surface, the sway velocity (23 mm/s) was about three times as great as in the control subjects (8 mm/s) (fig. 2). Vibration at higher frequencies increased successively the body sway reaching at 80 Hz an average sway velocity of 34 mm/s. The difference between the elderly subjects and the control subjects was statistically highly significant at all vibration frequencies and in the baseline values ($p < 0.001$).

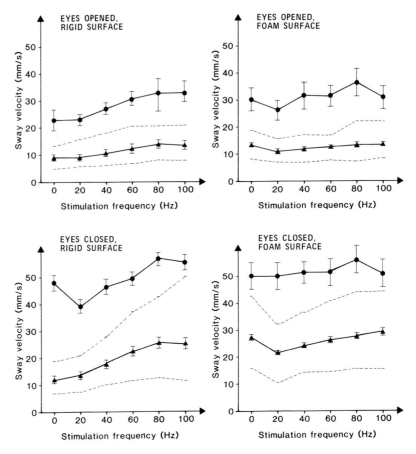

Fig. 2. Posturography results in elderly subjects (●) and control subjects (▲) at different visual and support surface conditions. Means and standard errors of means are given. Shaded area indicates 95% confidence interval for normal body sway velocities.

Rigid Surface without Visual Control

The postural control was severely deteriorated when the oldest old stood on the rigid surface without visual control (fig. 2). In the quiet stance the average sway velocity was 48 mm/s and exceeded the normal values (11 mm/s) by a factor of four. Exposure to vibration at 20 Hz caused a stabilizing effect for the posture. At higher frequencies vibration only slightly increased the body sway and at 80 Hz an average sway velocity of 51 mm/s was reached. In the oldest olds no significant differences were found between the different frequencies of vibration and baseline value. Nevertheless, the oldest olds differed highly significantly from control subjects at all stimulation frequencies and at baseline values (p <0.001). The Romberg quotient was 0.48 for the oldest olds, which contrasted with 0.71 observed in control subjects.

Foam Rubber Covered Surface in Visual Control Condition

With eyes open the oldest olds displayed almost identical body sway on foam rubber covered surface as on the rigid surface. Thus, during baseline conditions the sway velocity averaged 30 mm/s and reached a vibration frequency of 80 Hz at an average sway velocity of 36 mm/s.

In the oldest olds no significant differences between the different vibration frequencies and baseline values were observed. Furthermore, no differences were observed in the test where the oldest olds stood on a bare surface and a foam rubber covered surface (fig. 2). When compared with the control subjects on the foam rubber covered surface, throughout the test, the oldest old displayed sway velocities twice as high; this difference was statistically highly significant (p <0.001).

Foam Rubber Covered Surface without Visual Control

With eyes closed on the foam rubber covered surface the sway velocity averaged 50 mm/s during baseline conditions. Exposure to vibration produced almost no increase in body sway velocity (fig. 2). The body sway on the foam rubber covered surface did not differ from that measured on rigid surface in non-visual conditions. Nevertheless, at all stimulation frequencies and at baseline measurements the oldest olds had about 4 times higher sway velocity than the control subjects, a difference that was statistically highly significant (p <0.001).

Discussion

In the present study we evaluated the postural stability in the oldest olds during different postural control conditions. During the test the calf muscles were exposed to local vibration. This stimulation activated the muscle spindles and Golgi tendon organs and caused vibration-induced body sway. The extent of body sway in the present study describes the role of functional stretch reflexes triggered by calf muscles during postural destabilization. The activation of the functional stretch reflex during vibration was rather vague when compared with the control subjects or with patients with vestibular deficits [Pyykkö et al., 1986a]. When the subject was placed on a foam rubber covered surface in visual control conditions no further destabilization in postural stance was observed. Since the foam rubber covered surface effectively blocks the pressoreceptor influx from the soles the results indicate that the elderly subjects have a poor postural control also with pressoreceptor influx from the sole. Thus, the relative shortages of postural influx by proprioceptive and exteroceptive influx together with the absence of tendon reflexes and with defective vibration sensation is indicative of peripheral polyneuropathy in the oldest olds.

During life the hierarchy between the receptor system for postural control is plastic, i.e. a child is more dependent on proprioceptive and vestibular cues than visual cues [Sheldon, 1963]. Adults tend to trust more in visual cues than in vestibular and proprioceptive ones as was also observed in this study. The oldest olds controlled their posture almost entirely by visual influx. Thus, closure of the eyes, whether on a bare surface or a foam rubber covered surface, increased the sway velocity by a factor of two, which contrasted with results from the control subjects. Thus, the oldest olds had an enhancement of visual control of about 30% when compared with control subjects.

Since, in the present study, the stretch reflexes and functional stretch reflexes were defective in the elderly subject, the postural control during sudden falls and slips cannot be accurate. The weight of the postural control was put on the visual control system. The visual system is, however, slow and can control the posture at a latency of 120–200 ms, which is far too long a time interval to prevent falls and provide adequate landing response. Thus, for the prevention of accidental falls the floor should be kept even, since once a misstep occurs a fall may not be controlled by the postural mechanisms.

References

Aalto, H.; Pyykkö, I.; Starck, J.: Computerized posturography. A development of measuring system. Acta oto-lar. suppl. (in press 1988).

Barlett, S.A.; Maki, B.E.; Fernie, G.R.; Holliday, P.J.; Gryfe, C.I.: On the classification of a geriatric subject as a faller or nonfaller. Med. biol. Eng. Comp. *24:* 219–222 (1986).

Bauer, G.C.H.: Epidemiology of fractures; in Barzel, Osteoporosis (Grune & Stratton, New York 1970).

Diener, H.C.; Dichgans, J.; Guschlbauer, B.; Mau, H.: The significance of proprioception on postural stabilization as assessed by ischemia. Brain Res. *296:* 103–109 (1984).

Droulez, J.; Berthoz, A.A.; Vidal, P.P.: Use and limits of visual vestibular interaction in the control of posture; in Igarashi, Black, Vestibular and visual control on posture and locomotor equilibrium. 7th Int. Symp. Int. Soc. Posturography, Houston 1983, pp. 14–21 (Karger, Basel 1985).

Era, P.: Sensory, psychomotor and motor functions in men of different ages. Scand. J. soc. Med. suppl. 39 (1987).

Eyzaguirre, C.; Fidone, S.J.: Physiology of the nervous system; 2nd ed., pp. 163–248 (Year Book, Chicago 1975).

Holliday, P.J.; Fernie, G.R.: Postural sway during low frequency floor oscillation in young and elderly subjects; in Igarashi, Black, Vestibular and visual control on posture and locomotor equilibrium. 7th Int. Symp. Int. Soc. Posturography, Houston 1983, pp. 66–69 (Karger, Basel 1985).

Overstall, P.W.; Exton-Smith, A.N.; Imms, F.J.; Johnson, A.L.: Falls in the elderly related to postural imbalance. Br. med. J. i: 261–264 (1977).

Pyykkö, I.; Starck, J.; Scholtz, H.-J.; Meyer, E.; Aalto, H.; Enebom, H.: Evaluation of vestibular deficiency using posturography; in Claussen, Kirtane, Vertigo, nausea, tinnitus and hearing loss in cardio-vascular diseases, pp. 363–370 (Elsevier, Amsterdam 1986a).

Pyykkö, I.; Toppila, E.; Starck, J.; Aalto, H.; Enebom, H.; Seidel, H.: Computerized posturography: development of stimulus and analysis methods; in Claussen, Kirtane, Vertigo, nausea, tinnitus and hearing loss in cardio-vascular diseases, pp. 353–362 (Elsevier, Amsterdam 1986b).

Sheldon, J.H.: The effect of age on the control of sway. Geront. clin. 5: 129–138 (1963).

Waller, J.A.: Falls among the elderly — human and environmental factors. Accid. Anal. Prev. 10: 31–33 (1978).

Ilmari Pyykkö, MD, Department of Otolaryngology, University Hospital of Helsinki, Haartmaninkatu 2-4 E, SF-00290 Helsinki (Finland)

Adv. Oto-Rhino-Laryn., vol. 41, pp. 152–161 (Karger, Basel 1988)

Development of Righting Reflexes, Gross Motor Functions and Balance in Infants with Labyrinth Hypoactivity with or without Mental Retardation

K. Kaga, H. Maeda, J. Suzuki

Department of Otolaryngology, Teikyo University School of Medicine, Kaga Itabshi-ku, Tokyo, Japan

In infants and children with congenital or acquired hypoactive labyrinths, impairment of postural control is common and the development of gross motor functions in the acquisition of head control, sitting and walking is delayed [6], but fine motor function is usually preserved unless disorders of the central nervous system are present [4]. These children eventually catch up with normals because multisensory innervation and motor systems compensate for the deficit, but the length of the delay in acquiring normal gross motor skills and the final acquisition of motor skills and balance functions are controversial issues [4, 6, 9].

It has been pointed out that vestibular impairment is likely to be found in children with severe or profound hearing loss since the vestibular end organ and cochlea are closely related in their anatomy [1, 10, 11] and ontogeny and may be affected by the same embryological or noxious factors, for example, viral or bacterial infection [7].

As the vestibular reflexes of infants are not comparable to those of adults, it is particularly important in the evaluation of young deaf patients that their vestibular function and gross motor function should be assessed with reference to that of their age-mates [2, 3, 6].

The present investigation had as its primary objective the longitudinal study of patients with congenital and acquired vestibular hypofunction or afunction as these conditions relate to delayed acquisition of gross motor function or reacquisition of gross motor function and balance.

To accomplish this, we first obtained quantitative data on the development of these skills in normal infants and children, along with measures of the maturation of their vestibular responses to the damped-rotation test [6]. We then compared these data with those of infants and children with congenital and acquired deafness and with or without mental retardation relating degree of vestibular impairment to delay in reaching milestones of gross motor development. We chose patients who were demonstrated to have a marked decrease of vestibular responses.

Methods

Subjects

Thirty-three infants and children with profound hearing loss and vestibular hypoactivity were studied for the development of righting gross motor functions and balance. These cases were classified into three major groups (I–III), which were subdivided into two minor groups (A: normal intelligence; B: mental retardation). Group IA: Eight infants who had congenital hearing loss, normal intelligence, and were without inner ear anomalies; group IB: 7 infants who had congenital hearing loss, mental retardation, and were without inner ear anomalies. Group IIA: Four infants with normal intelligence who had inner ear anomalies demonstrated by computed tomography (CT) of the temporal bones; group IIB: 4 infants who had inner ear anomalies and mental retardation. Group IIIA: Five without mental retardation who had lost labyrinthine function after meningitis in childhood; group IIIB: 5 with mental retardation who had lost labyrinthine function after miningitis or measles encephalitis.

Procedures

Auditory Function Test. The hearing loss of these infants was assessed by behavioral audiometry or conditioned orientation reflex audiometry and auditory brain stem responses (ABR) [5]. The ABR for 85 dB HL click stimuli were absent in these cases.

Vestibular Function Test. Cooperative patients were tested for vestibular dysfunction by ice water caloric test. However, because caloric stimulation is generally unsatisfactory in infants or mentally retarded children, vestibular function was assessed by means of the damped-rotation test. Electrodes were applied just lateral to both eyes to record horizontal eye movements, and the subject was held on the mother's lap in a rotating chair. The chair was then accelerated to a maximum rotational velocity of 200°/s, maximum acceleration being 300°/s. Velocity then decreased to 0° over a period of 20 s with approximately six revolutions. The test was conducted twice, for clockwise and counterclockwise rotation. Electronystagmography (ENG) responses were recorded by a time constant, 0.003 s, and scored according to duration and number of beats of perotatory nystagmus. These measures are more practical than slow phase velocity, since young children cannot cooperate in the calibration procedure required for accurate velocity measurements. Normal values have been reported previously [6]. In these cases, either ice water caloric tests or damped-rotation tests revealed no responses or very poor ones.

Righting reflex and gross motor function were evaluated by Eviatar's neurovestibular examination of infants and children and development milestones of gross motor function, which were observed for head control, sitting, crawling, and walking [2]. After walking was attained, Romberg position, standing and locomotion on balance beam, and standing on one foot were used to evaluate balance function.

Results

Group IA (congenital deafness and vestibular hypofunction with normal intelligence and without inner ear anomalies): Eight patients' age of acquisition of gross motor functions are shown in table I. In table II, motor skills and balance functions of a typical case acquired at the age of 6 years are presented with a brief case history.

Group IB (congenital deafness and vestibular hypofunction with mental retardation and without inner ear anomalies): Seven patients' age of acquisition of gross motor functions are shown in table I. Each age of acquisition in this group was later than in group IA.

Group IIA (congenital deafness and vestibular hypofunction with inner ear anomalies and normal intelligence): Four patients' age of acquisition of gross motor functions are shown in table III. Type-1 inner ear anomalies indicate absence of cochlea and semicircular canals, type-2 absence of all semicircular canals only, and type-3 absence of lateral semicircular canals only. In figure 1, CT of a type-1 case is shown. Each age of acquisition in this group was close to that in group IA.

Group IIB (congenital deafness and vestibular hypofunction with inner ear anomalies and mental retardation): Four patients' age of acquisition of gross motor functions are shown in table III. Each age of acquisition in this group was later than that in group IIA and close to that in group IB.

Group IIIA (acquired deafness and vestibular hypofunction with normal intelligence): Four patients' age of acquisition of gross motor functions and balance after loss of labyrinthine function due to meningitis are shown in table IV. The course of 2 cases after loss of labyrinthine function due to meningitis is illustrated in figure 2. These 2 cases suggest that gross motor functions and balance could be lost at once and acquired again if the age of loss of labyrinthine function was around one year.

Group IIIB (acquired deafness and vestibular hypofunction with mental retardation): Four patients' gross motor functions after loss of labyrinthine functions are shown in table IV. Each age of acquisition in this group was seriously later than in any other group.

Table I. Group IA: Congenital deafness with normal intelligence

Case	Age	Head control	Crawling	Sitting	Standing with support	Walking
1	1 y 9 m	6 m	9 m	9 m	9 m	1 y 6 m
2	2 y	7 m	7 m	9 m	?	1 y 5 m
3	2 y 1 m	6 m	9 m	9 m	1 y 1 m	1 y 8 m
4	3 y 0 m	6 m	12 m	11 m	1 y 4 m	2 y 0 m
5	3 y 1 m	4 m	7 m	7 m	10 m	1 y 10 m
6	4 y 7 m	8 m	?	1 y 3 m	?	2 y 0 m
7	4 y 11 m	6 m	1 y 2 m	8 m	12 m	2 y 1 m
8	6 y	5 m	8 m	12 m	7 m	2 y 3 m
Range[a]		4–8 m	7 m–1 y 2 m	8 m–1 y 3 m	9 m–1 y 4 m	1 y 5 m–2 y 3 m
X̄		6 m	9.4 m	10 m	11.5 m	1 y 10 m
SD		1.2	2.6	2.6	2.7	3.5

Group IB: Congenital deafness with mental retardation

Case	Age	Head	Crawling	Sitting	Standing with support	Walking	Remarks
1	1 y 2 m	9 m	1 y 0 m	1 y 2 m	1 y 3 m		cytomegalovirus
2	2 y	12 m	1 y 5 m	1 y 4 m	1 y 4 m	2 y 5 m	toe anomaly
3	4 y	10 m	?	1 y 1 m	3 y 2 m	3 y 4 m	cytomegalovirus
4	6 y	6 m	2 y 4 m	1 y 4 m	1 y 11 m	4 y	cytomegalovirus
5	6 y 1 m	4 m	?	?	(–)		ventricular dilation
6	7 y	16 m	?	3 y 0 m	?	4 y	low height
7	8 y	12 m	1 y 10 m	2 y 0 m	2 y 7 m	3 y 5 m	hyperkinetic
Range[a]		4–16 m	12 m–2 y 4 m	1 y 2 m–3 y 0 m	1 y 3 m–3 y 2 m	2–4 y	
[a]Normal range		3–4 m	7–10 m	6–8 m	10–11 m	10–12m	

Table II. Case S.O.: female, born 1976

Birth weight:	3,375 g, full-term
Perinatal accident:	n.p.; family history: n.p.
Age at first visit:	10 months
Chief complaints:	(1) floppiness; (2) deafness
Audiological tests:	COR — no responses at 100 dB
	ABR — no responses at 85 dB
Vestibular tests:	no nystagmus to the rotation test
	no vestibular righting response
	remarkable hypotonus without pyramidal signs

Motor milestones	Attainment	Normal range
1 Head control	5 months	(2–3 months)
2 Crawling	8 months	(7–10 months)
3 Sitting	12 months	(6–8 months)
4 Standing with support	9 months	(10–11 months)
5 Initial walk	2 years and 3 months	(10–12 months)

Acquired motor skills at age of 6 years	
Fine motor	normal
Gross motor	
(a) Walking	normal with eyes open and covered
(b) On balance beam	normal with eyes open and covered
(c) Running	normal
(d) Romberg position	normal with eyes open and covered
(e) Standing on one foot	impaired with eyes open and covered
(f) Hopping on one foot	skillful with eyes open and covered
(g) Sports	baseball, gymnastics

Discussion

Our data provide further evidence for the thesis that vestibular dysfunction may delay the achievement of gross motor functions and balance in infants and children, whether the cause is congenital or acquired.

It is clear that impairment or absence of the labyrinthine righting reflex was associated with delay of gross motor landmarks and balance functions in these children but that the children were able to acquire these skills eventually, provided that mental retardation and neurological disorders were not also present.

In early childhood the vestibulospinal reflex helps to maintain postural control while the visuomotor and somatosensory systems of the central

Table III. Group IIA: Inner ear anomalies in cases with normal intelligence

Case	Age	Type of inner ear anomaly	Head control	Crawling	Sitting	Standing with support	Walking
1	4 y	I	7 m	10 m	11 m	1 y 8 m	2 y
2	7 y	II	4 m	8 m	10 m	9 m	1 y 10 m
3	7 y	II	4 m	2 y	1 y 6 m	2 y	2 y 9 m
4	13 y	III	3 m	7 m	6 m	10 m	12 m
Range[a]			3–7 m	8 m–2 y	6 m–1 y 6 m	9 m–1 y 8 m	12 m–2 y 9 m

Group IIB: Inner ear anomalies in cases with mental retardation

Case	Age	Type	Head control	Crawling	Sitting	Standing with support	Walking
1	1 y 5 m	I	1 y 1 m	1 y 3 m	1 y 2 m	(–)	(–)
2	2 y 1 m	II	8 m	(–)	1 y 10 m	(–)	(–)
3	8 y	II	2 y	2 y 6 m	3 y	3 y	3 y 6 m
4	10 y	II	1 y 6 m	?	?	2 y 3 m	4 y 6 m
Range[a]			8 m–2 y	1 y 3 m–2 y 6 m	1 y 2 m–3 y	2 y 3 m–3 y	3 y 6 m–4 y 6 m
[a]Normal range			3–4 m	7–10 m	6–8 m	10–11 m	10–12 m

nervous system are developing [12]. Therefore, labyrinthine function is important in the development of balance and locomotion. It follows that impairment of the righting reflex in infancy may lead to delayed achievement of gross motor milestones because of impairment of labyrinthine muscle tone and neck or extremity reflexes as well as to decreased balance [4, 5, 8].

However, the delay seems to be readily compensated for by the plasticity of the central nervous system and the development of the proprioceptive, visual, and motor systems [12]. As compensation in later childhood is quite good, special tests should be applied for older children to elicit any gait abnormality due to vestibular dysfunction. For that purpose, standing on one foot with the eyes either open or covered is recommended to detect vestibular dysfunction, because it is a sensitive test of balance dysfunction and is not easily compensated for even in adolescence. Fine motor skills are not delayed in these patients, partly because labyrinthine reflexes must be

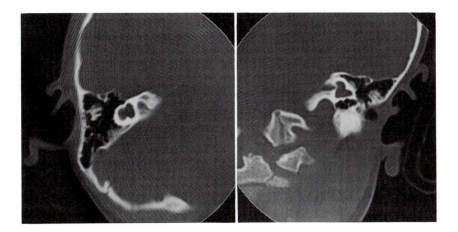

Fig. 1. Computed tomography of temporal bones in a 4-year-old boy. Cochlea and all semicircular canals are absent in this case, but the vestibulum is formed like a large cyst. This is case 1 of group IIA in table III.

Table IV. Group IIIA: Acquired deafness with normal intelligence

Case	Age	Onset	Neurological signs after meningitis
1	2 y 2 m	11 m	loss of head control and balance
2	1 y 7 m	1 y 1 m	loss of head control and balance
3	4 y	2 y 2 m	vestibular ataxia over 3 months
4	5 y	4 y 6 m	vestibular ataxia over 2 months
5	10 y	9 y	vestibular ataxia over 2 months

Group IIIB: Acquired deafness with mental retardation

Case	Age	Onset	Head control	Crawling	Sitting	Standing with support	Walking	Remarks
1	12 m	0 m	—	—	—	—	—	meningitis
2	9 m	4 m	—	—	—	—	—	meningitis
3	1 y 6 m	7 m	—	—	—	—	—	meningitis
4	7 y	1 y 1 m	7 m	1 y 6 m	10 m	3 y	—	measles
5	4 y	1 y 9 m	4 m	6 m	?	2 y 5 m	2 y 5 m	meningitis
Normal range			3–4 m	7–10 m	6–8 m	10–11 m	10–12 m	

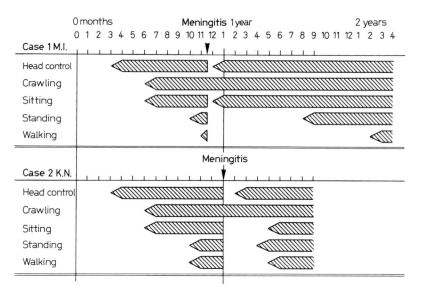

Fig. 2. The course of 2 cases after loss of labyrinthine function due to meningitis. The shaded area indicates the acquisition period for each gross motor function. Case 1 lost vestibular function at the age of 11 months and gross motor functions except for crawling disappeared but were acquired again. Case 2 lost vestibular functions at the age of one year and one month, and gross motor functions, except for crawling, disappeared but were acquired again.

controlled by voluntary movements of the higher functions. However, if these patients have accompanying mental retardation, even without other neurological signs, the acquisition of gross motor functions and balance can be seriously delayed, probably because of slow central compensation, slow association of multiple sensory inputs and/or slow motor learning.

References

1   Arnvig, J.: Vestibular function in deafness and severe hardness of hearing. Acta oto-lar. *45:* 283–288 (1955).
2   Eviatar, L.; Eviatar, A.: Neurovestibular examination of infants and children. Adv. Oto-Rhino-Laryng., vol. 23, pp. 169–191 (Karger, Basel 1978).
3   Eviatar, L.; Miranda, S.; Eviatar, A.; Freeman, K.; Borkowski, M.: Development of nystagmus in response to vestibular stimulation in infants. Ann. Neurol. *5:* 508–514 (1979).

4   Horiuchi, M.; Kaga, K.; Tanaka, Y.: Development of gross and fine motor functions in infants with profound hearing loss. Audiol. Jap. *28:* 709–716 (1985).
5   Kaga, K.; Tanaka, Y.: Auditory brainstem response and behavioral audiometry. Archs Otolar. *106:* 564–566 (1980).
6   Kaga, K.; Suzuki, J.; Marsh, R.R.; Tanaka, Y.: Influence of labyrinthine hypoactivity on gross motor development of infants. Ann. N.Y. Acad. Sci. *374:* 412–420 (1981).
7   Kaplan, S.L.; Goddard, J.; Van Kleeck, et al.: Ataxia and deafness in children due to bacterial meningitis. Pediatrics *68:* 8–13 (1981).
8   Molina-Negro, P.; Bertrand, R.A.; Martin, E.; Gioani, A.: The role of the vestibular system in relation to muscle tone and postural reflexes in man. Acta oto-lar. *89:* 524–533 (1980).
9   Rapin, I.: Hypoactive labyrinths and motor development. Clin. Pediat. *13:* 922–937 (1974).
10 Swisher, L.P.; Gannon, R.P.: A comparison of auditory and vestibular responses in hearing-impaired children. Acta oto-lar. *66:* 89–96 (1968).
11 Sandberg, L.E.; Terkildsen, K.: Caloric tests in deaf children. Archs Otolar. *81:* 350–354 (1965).
12 Yakovlev, P.I.; Lecours, A.-R.: The myelogenetic cycles of regional maturation of the brain; in Minkowski, Regional development of the brain in early life, pp. 3–70 (Blackwell, Oxford 1967).

K. Kaga, MD, Department of Otolaryngology,
Teikyo University School of Medicine, Kaga 2-11-1, Itabashi-ku, Tokyo 173 (Japan)

Adv. Oto-Rhino-Laryng., vol. 41, pp. 162–165 (Karger, Basel 1988)

Otolithic Control of Posture: Vestibulo-Spinal Reflexes in a Patient with a Tullio Phenomenon

W. Fries, M. Dieterich, T. Brandt

Neurologische Universitätsklinik, Klinikum Grosshadern, München, FRG

Vestibulo-spinal reflexes in man have been studied in experiments using a sudden unexpected fall which evoked an early EMG response in the lower limb muscles with a latency of 60–80 ms [Melville-Jones and Watt, 1971; Greenwood and Hopkins, 1976], the early component depending — at least in cat — on the integrity of the vestibular apparatus [Watt, 1976]. Its functional significance has been seen in preparing the subject for landing. To what extent vestibular mechanisms are involved in the control of posture and gait is still debated controversially, since vestibular responses after perturbation of stance are reported to occur with a latency of some 180 ms [Nashner et al., 1982]. However, a response in the tib. ant. muscles probably of vestibular origin with a latency of about 60 ms is deduced if the time course of head acceleration is taken into account [Allum and Keshner, 1986].

The rare clinical condition of a Tullio phenomenon of the otolithic type [Brandt et al., 1988] in an otherwise healthy young man offered the opportunity to study directly the involvement of otolithic vestibulo-spinal reflexes in the control of posture. The patient, a professional horn player, experienced paroxysmal oscillopsia associated with an ocular tilt reaction (OTR) as well as postural imbalance and dizziness when his left ear was stimulated with loud sounds, particularly at frequencies around 490 ± 20 Hz. There is evidence that his symptoms are elicited by direct inadequate mechanical stimulation of the saccule and/or the utricle secondary to a loose hypermobile stapes footplate which is driven by the stapedius reflex [Brandt et al., 1988].

Effects of sound applied to the left ear of 490 ± 20 Hz and 95 dB (above hearing threshold) on postural stability were investigated by electromyo-

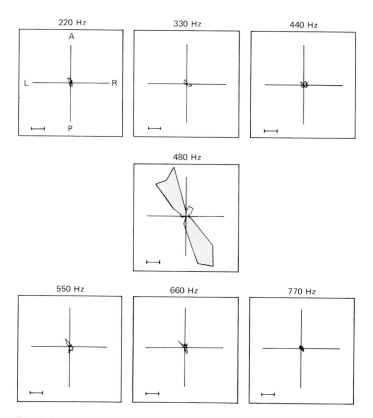

Fig. 1. Sway histogram of postural imbalance with a predominantly diagonal body sway evoked by sound of 480 Hz applied to the left ear, compared with almost normal sway histograms at other frequencies but same intensity. Calibration bar: 1 cm.

graphic and posturographic (Kistler platform) measurements. The EMG activity of the tib. ant. muscles and gastrocn. muscles of both legs was recorded with surface electrodes. The sound induced a destabilization of stance with a body sway predominantly from right and backward to left and forward (see sway histogram fig. 1), the initial response being to the right and backward. Subjectively, however, the patient experienced an initial sensation of falling towards the left and forward.

The EMG recordings revealed a co-activation of the ipsilateral lower leg muscles, following both the onset as well as the offset of the sound stimulus. After the initial phasic response which appeared more pronounced in the tib. ant. muscle, there was a tonic increase of activity as long as the sound was

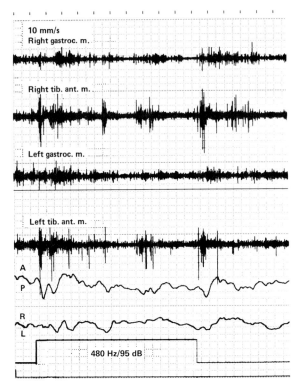

10 mm/s
Right gastroc. m.

Right tib. ant. m.

Left gastroc. m.

Left tib. ant. m.

A
P

R
L

480 Hz/95 dB

Fig. 2. Original EMG recording of lower leg muscles of both legs (top four traces) and recordings of Kistler platform. Note the activation both at onset and offset of sound (bottom trace).

present (fig. 2). The latencies ranged from about 47 to 80 ms for the ipsilateral tib. ant. muscle; the variation of latencies seemed to depend on habituation as well as the expectancy of the next stimulus. The gastrocn. muscle was found to be coactivated following the tib. ant. muscle with a delay of on average 5 ms. Responses in the contralateral leg occurred about 10 ms later. The body sway commenced as early as 80 ms after the onset of sound. Because of these short latencies, we have to assume a direct vestibulo-spinal mechanism for the postural imbalance after sound stimulation rather than a transcortical loop with compensatory body movements initiated by the change of graviceptive perception. When the sound stimulus was given while the patient was resting supine, no detectable EMG response was seen, even if there was a tonic level of discharge due to voluntary isometric contraction. Similarly, modifications of posture in which lower leg muscles were actually not involved in maintaning of posture, such as sitting or standing on one leg, were found to cancel otolithic muscle reflexes in tib. ant. and gastrocn. muscles.

We conclude, therefore, that otolithic evoked vestibulo-spinal reflexes have a fast as well as functionally significant influence on the control of upright stance in man via descending pathways. This direct (three-neuron arc?) sensorimotor link may be modified by the actual postural program such as standing, lying or sitting.

References

Allum, J.H.J.; Keshner, E.A.: Vestibular and proprioceptive control of sway stabilization; in Bles, Brandt, Disorders of posture and gait, pp. 19–40 (Elsevier, Amsterdam 1986).

Brandt, T.; Dieterich, M.; Fries, W.: Otolithic Tullio phenomenon typically presents as paroxysmal ocular tilt reaction. Adv. Oto-Rhino-Laryng., vol. 42, pp. 153–156 (Karger, Basel 1988).

Greenwood, R.; Hopkins, A.: Muscle responses during sudden falls in man. J. Physiol. *254:* 507–518 (1976).

Melville-Jones, G.; Watt, I.G.D.: Muscular control of landing from unexpected falls in man. J. Physiol. *219:* 729–737 (1971).

Nashner, L.M.; Black, F.O.; Wall, C., III: Adaptation to altered support and visual conditions during stance: patients with vestibular deficits. J. Neurosci. *2:* 536–544 (1982).

Watt, D.G.D.: Response of cats to sudden falls: an otolith-originating reflex assisting landing. J. Neurophysiol. *39:* 257–265 (1976).

Dr. W. Fries, PhD, Neurologische Universitätsklinik, Klinikum Grosshadern, Marchioninistrasse 15, D-8000 München 70 (FRG)

Adv. Oto-Rhino-Laryng., vol. 41, pp. 166–172 (Karger, Basel 1988)

The Examination of Body Sway in Normal Subjects and Patients with Ménière's Disease or Cerebellar Dysfunction

H. Ishizaki[a], *K. Umemura*[a], *H. Mineta*[a], *M. Nozue*[a], *I. Matsuoka*[b], *K. Iwasaki*[b], *Y. Nishida*[b]

[a]Department of Otorhinolaryngology, Hamamatsu University School of Medicine, Handa-cho, Hamamatsu; [b]Shizuoka General Hospital, Kita-ando, Shizuoka, Japan

Introduction

The body sway test is useful to evaluate patients with vertigo, especially to diagnose patients with unilateral Ménière's disease or cerebellar dysfunctions. The purpose of this paper is to investigate the origin of sway for each frequency range, analyzing the sway distance into X and Y components by using a moving average method in order to remove high frequency noise.

Materials and Methods

The subjects were 31 controls, 66 patients with unilateral Ménière's disease and 15 patients with cerebellar dysfunctions. They stood still on the gravicorder for 30 s with eyes open and closed. Simultaneous recording was made on the magnetic tape for a further computer analysis. We carried out frequency analysis after dividing the whole frequency into 3 ranges from 0.033 to 2.95 Hz. We adopted a 'moving five point average method', correcting each point by averaging the consecutive five points with the sample in the middle.

Figure 1 shows our analysis system. We analyzed the data stored in the recorder about distances and frequencies with a signal processor. The data contained many noises, including high frequency noises beyond our physiological range. Therefore, we eliminated the high frequency noises by using the technique of 'moving five point average'.

Figure 2 shows our method. This was the best method to eliminate high frequency noises. We examined the frequency range between 0.033 and 2.95 Hz.

Figure 3 shows the power spectrum divided into 3 ranges at 0.5–1.0 Hz. The first peak was usually between 0.033 andf 0.5 Hz. We analyzed the frequency in X and Y components measured by relative numerical values.

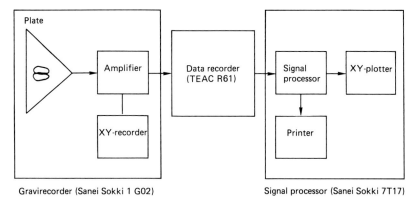

Fig. 1. Diagram of the gravirecorder and analysis system.

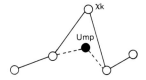

$$U_{mp} = \frac{1}{m} \sum_{P-\frac{(m-1)}{2}}^{P+\frac{(m+1)}{2}} Xk$$

0.033 Hz < Moving average 5 < 2.95 Hz

Fig. 2. Moving average 5.

Results and Discussion

The two upper figures show the distances in X and Y components and directions of body sway in regression lines in 31 normal controls (fig. 4). There was no correlation between X and Y components with eyes open. The distance of body sway in the X direction was always longer than that of the Y direction, especially with eyes closed. The frequency analysis showed almost no difference with eyes open or closed. In the frequency range of 0.5 to 1.0 Hz, the body sway, if any, was a little more prominent with eyes closed [1]. The body sway consisted mainly of slow movements below 0.5 Hz. The Y

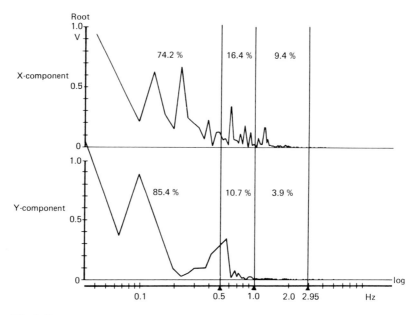

Fig. 3. Power spectrum.

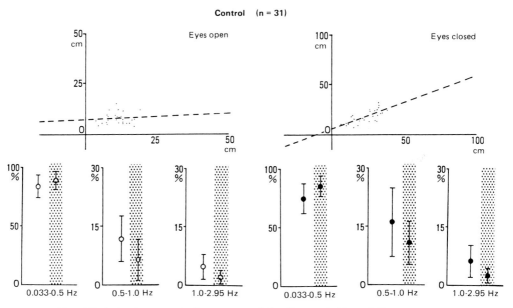

Fig. 4. Relation between the frequency and the distance in X- and Y-components.

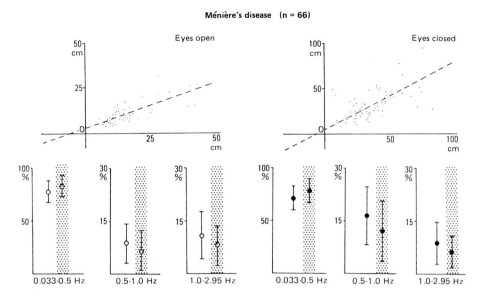

Fig. 5. Relation between the frequency and the distance in X- and Y-components.

component of body sway below 0.5 Hz was dominant (p $<$0.05). The X component in 0.5 to 2.95 Hz was more significant than the Y component both with eyes open and closed [2].

From the results of the relation between the directional distance analysis and frequency analysis in X and Y components, it was suggested that the direction of body sway consisted in the frequency over 0.5 Hz. The data obtained from 66 patients with unilateral Ménière's disease are shown in figure 5.

The distance of body sway in the X direction was always longer than in the Y direction. But the regression lines showed that the Y component was more eminent with eyes closed. The frequency analysis showed almost the same pattern as those in normal controls, but more eminent in the range between 0.5 and 2.95 Hz.

Ikegami [3] also reported that the frequency below 0.5 Hz occupied the most part. The frequency over 0.5 Hz in the X component was more significant than the Y component.

The relation between directional distance analysis and frequency analysis in X and Y components was observed over 0.5 Hz. Right and left sway was notable in the patient with unilateral loss of labyrinthine function [4].

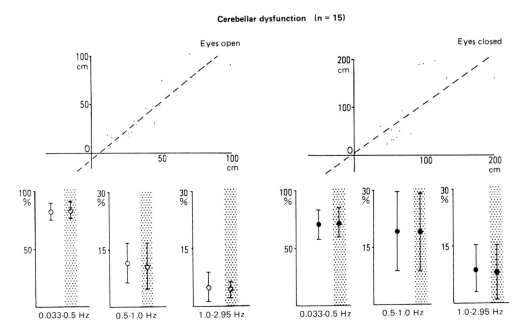

Fig. 6. Relation between the frequency and the distance in X- and Y-components.

It was suggested that the frequency over 0.5 Hz was mainly vestibular control [2].

The data from 15 patients with cerebellar dysfunctions including spino-cerebellar degeneration are shown in figure 6. From the regression lines, the distance of body sway in the Y direction was more eminent than in normal controls and the patients with unilateral Ménière's disease [5]. The frequency analysis showed no significant difference between X and Y components in each range [2].

The body sway was mainly composed of slow movements below 0.5 Hz. The frequency in 0.5–1.0 Hz was more eminent with eyes closed, and also between 1.0 and 2.95 Hz [6]. Figure 7 shows the summation of the frequency analysis of the preceding 3 cases. The slow movements below 0.5 Hz occupied most of the body sway.

The Y component of body sway below 0.5 Hz was dominant in normal controls and also in patients with Ménière's disease [1, 2]. However, this was not observed in patients with cerebellar dysfunctions. The frequency of body sway in 0.5–1.0 Hz in 3 cases was more significant in diversity with eyes closed than with eyes open.

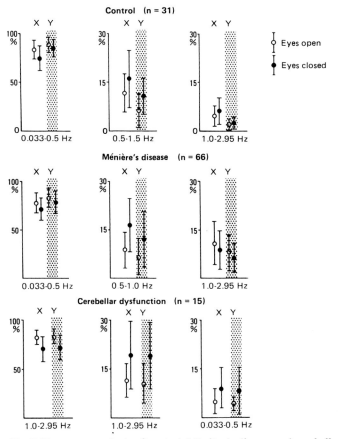

Fig. 7. Frequency analysis of control, Ménière's disease and cerebellar dysfunction.

The X component of body sway in 0.5–1.0 Hz was greater than the Y component in normal controls and the patients with Ménière's disease. However, it was not the case in patients with cerebellar dysfunctions. This was more significant in patients with unilateral Ménière's disease between 1.0 and 2.95 Hz.

It was suggested that the predominance of the X component originated in the vestibular function. The whole direction of body sway was determined by sway over 0.5 Hz. From these data, the body sway below 0.5 Hz did not originate in vestibular function. If we consider that the mechanism of body sway involves the cerebellar and vestibular networks, it may be said that the body sway below 0.5 Hz was regulated by the cerebellar function.

References

1   Yoneda, S.; Tokumasu, K.: Frequency analysis of the movement of the center of gravity in normal upright standing. The influences of vision and different foot-forms. Equilibrium Res. *41:* 55–60 (1982).

2   Yoneda, S.; Tokumasu, K.: Frequency analysis of body sway in standing upright. Statistical study in the cases of peripheral vestibular disease and central nervous disturbance. Equilibrium Res. *43:* 264–271 (1984).

3   Ikegami, A.: Study on amplitude and velocity of movement of the center of gravity in Romberg's posture. Aging changes and diagnostic value. Otolaryng. Jap. *86:* 886–898 (1983).

4   Tokita, T.; Maeda, M.; Miyata, H.: The role of the labyrinth in standing posture regulation. Acta oto-lar. *91:* 521–527 (1983).

5   Dichgans, J.; Diener, H.C.: Postural ataxia in late atrophy of the cerebellar anterior lobe and its differential diagnosis; in Igarashi, Black, Vestibular control on posture and locomotion, pp. 282–289 (Karger, Basel 1983).

6   Diener, H.C.; Dichgans, J.; Bacher, M.; Gompf, B.: Quantification of postural sway in normals and patients with cerebellar disease. Electroenceph. clin. Neurophysiol. *57:* 134–142 (1984).

H. Ishizaki, MD, Department of Otorhinolaryngology, Hamamatsu University
School of Medicine, 3600 Handa-cho, Hamamatsu 431-31 (Japan)

Adv. Oto-Rhino-Laryn., vol. 41, pp. 173–178 (Karger, Basel 1988)

Behavior of the Vestibulo-Ocular Reflex at High Rotational Velocities in the Rhesus Monkey

R.D. Tomlinson

Department of Otolaryngology, Physiology and the Playfair Neuroscience Unit, University of Toronto, Toronto, Canada

Introduction

In order for gaze stability to be maintained following the saccadic portion of a combined eye-head gaze shift, the vestibulo-ocular reflex (VOR) or some other mechanism must generate a compensatory eye movement during the terminal portion of the head movement, after the eye has arrived on target. This compensatory roll-back of the eyes has been widely assumed to be vestibular in origin [1]. As monkeys are known to generate head movements in excess of 1,200°/s [3], it seems difficult to imagine how the VOR could possibly compensate for such high velocities especially as the VOR has been shown to saturate at about 350°/s in humans [2].

The present experiments were designed to investigate this question in more detail. As the only data currently available on the upper velocity limits of the VOR is in humans [2], we wished to discover whether or not such a limit also existed in rhesus monkeys. At the same time, we planned to look at the gaze changes that occurred during these high velocity rotations so that we could compare the eye trajectories with those we observed during active head movements.

Methods

Experiments were performed in 2 juvenile rhesus monkeys. eye and head position were both monitored with search coils using a phase-type coil system manufactured by CNC Engineering (Seattle). Gaze, head, and target position data were digitized on-line with a 2-ms sample interval and stored on magnetic tape for further analysis. Analyzed parameters were stored in a separate file.

High rotational velocities were obtained by having the experimenter suddenly rotate the chair as quickly as he was able by pulling on a lever on the rotating table to which the chair was attached. Springs were attached to the table so that it would oscillate in a quasisinusoidal fashion. In addition, the springs greatly increased the peak velocities which could be obtained. All rotations were carried out in a lighted room while the experimenter talked quietly to the animal. In this way we were able to achieve very high velocities without the monkey becoming frightened.

Results

Saccades during Passive Rotations

When the animals were manually rotated, we were able to achieve velocities of up to 900 °/s. The chair motion was roughly sinusoidal in nature with a frequency of approximately 1.5 Hz. The resulting nystagmus exhibited many long and slow saccades (fig. 1) where eye velocity was often negligible or was even seen to be reversed relative to the direction of gaze movement. We attempted to discover whether such slow saccades might be related to concurrent head velocity as would be expected if the slow eye movements were due to a summation of saccade and vestibular commands. This was done by measuring the head velocity at the time that eye-in-head velocity became zero even though a gaze saccade was in progress. There was no apparent correlation. In addition, these slow eye movements were not the result of the eye being driven to its mechanical limits as the orbital position where eye velocity became zero was found to often be close to primary position. Finally, although concurrent head velocity tended to be high, it was observed to be as low as 100°/s on occasion.

Somewhat surprisingly, however, both eye amplitude, E, and average velocity, $\dot{E}a$, were found to be related to the initial eye position; i.e. the position of the eye in the orbit prior to the initiation of the gaze saccade. Figures 2a and b illustrate this phenomenon for rightward (positive direction) gaze saccades. As the initial eye position moves in the direction of the gaze saccade, both the amplitude and velocity are seen to decrease until they both become negative for initial eye positions greater than 20° right. Thus, the change in eye position during the gaze saccade will tend to keep the eye within about 20° of the primary position, independent of the change in gaze angle. For any given desired change in gaze angle, the contribution of the eye to that change will be a function of the position of the eye in the orbit just prior to the initiation of the gaze saccade.

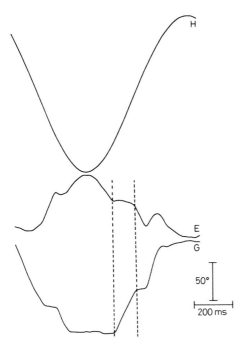

Fig. 1. Illustration of a gaze saccade with low eye velocity executed during high velocity passive whole body rotation; curves labelled E, H, and G represent eye, head and gaze (= E+H) position respectively. The two vertical dashed lines show the beginning and end of the saccade. In spite of the low eye velocity, the eye is not close to its rotational limits.

VOR Gain

When eye velocity was measured during the slow phase and plotted against concurrent head velocity, the results illustrated in figure 3 were obtained. Clearly, there is no evidence for saturation of the monkey VOR up to head velocities in excess of 800°/s. Although some upper limit must exist we were unable to generate high enough velocities to reach that limit.

In these same animals, the maximum observed saccadic velocity was 1,150°/s and this was only observed rarely. Most saccades exhibited peak velocities below 900°/s. Thus there was little or no difference between the eye velocities attained during saccades and those which resulted from vestibular stimulation.

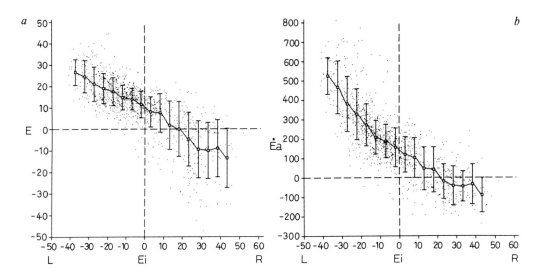

Fig. 2. Graphs of E (*a*) and Ėa (*b*) versus initial eye position. Note the decrease both E and Ėa as the initial position of the eye moves in the direction of the gaze saccade.

Conclusions

Previous authors have shown that the human VOR exhibits a soft saturation at about 350 °/s [2], well below the maximum saccadic velocities observed in the same subjects. The results described here indicate that the uper limits of the monkey VOR extend well beyond the above value, up to at least 900 °/s. As the same animals were observed to make saccadic eye movements which only rarely exceeded 900 °/s, it seems reasonable to assume that rhesus monkeys are able to make vestibular eye movements up to the limits imposed by the dynamic capabilities of the plant. This is a somewhat surprising observation in that humans exhibit such different behavior. It should be emphasized that the presence of many slow, or even reversed, eye movements during the gaze saccades makes the differentiation between vestibular and saccadic eye movements very difficult without reference to a gaze channel.

We found the behavior of gaze saccades executed during times of high rotational velocity unexpected. Specifically, the contribution of the eye to the

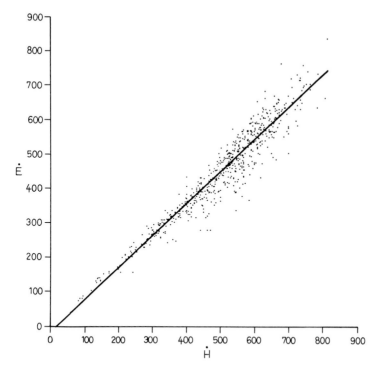

Fig. 3. Plot of eye velocity versus head velocity during slow phase eye movements. The slope of the regression line (0.92) is the mean reflex gain.

actual change in gaze position was found to be a function of the position of the eye in the orbit just prior to the initiation of the gaze saccade. Thus, on average, the eye moved towards a central location, independent of the direction of the saccade. If the eye started out deviated opposite to the direction of the quick phase, then the eye was seen to move in the same direction as the gaze change. If, however, the eye was already deviated in the direction of the gaze saccade, then the eye was often seen to move counter to the direction of gaze movement. Thus it would appear that the relative contributions of the eye and head to the change in gaze angle are not fixed but instead are systematically changed according to the orbital position of the eye just prior to the movement.

References

1   Bizzi, E.: ; Kalil, R.E.; Tagliasco, V.: Eye-head coordination in monkeys: evidence for centrally patterned organization. Science *173:* 452–454 (1971)

2   Pulaski, P.D.; Zee, D.S.; Robinson, D.A.: The behavior of the vestibulo-ocular reflex at high velocities of head rotation. Brain Res. *222:* 159-165 (1981).

3   Tomlinson, R.D.; Bahra, P.S.: Combined eye-head gaze shifts in the primate. I. Metrics. J. Neurophysiol. *56:* 1542–1557 (1986).

R.D. Tomlinson, MD, Department of Otolaryngology, Physiology and the Playfair Neuroscience Unit, University of Toronto, Toronto (Canada)

Adv. Oto-Rhino-Laryn., vol. 41, pp. 179–183 (Karger, Basel 1988)

Analysis of Vestibulo-Ocular Reflex Using Sweep Frequency Active Head Movements

Dennis P. O'Leary, Linda L. Davis, Geli-Ann Kitsigianis

Department of Otolaryngology, Head and Neck Surgery; University of Southern California School of Medicine, Los Angeles, Calif., USA

Introduction

The vestibulo-ocular reflex (VOR) is often stimulated by active head movements in the 2- to 6-Hz range during daily behavior [1]. But VOR rotational chair testing in this range is seldom done, requiring specialized, powerful rotational systems applied only recently [2–4].

Alternatively, use of active head movements as motion stimuli has the practical advantage that higher-frequency VOR analysis can be done by attaching lightweight eye and head movement sensors to a headstrap worn by the subject [5, 6]. A computer then records and analyzes the head movement stimuli and the eye movement responses. Our laboratory developed a vestibular autorotation test (VAT) as a new method of sweep-frequency VOR testing, based on 18 s of active head movements that increase linearly in frequency from 2 to 6 Hz [6, 7].

This report demonstrates the repeatability of the VAT, with multiple testing of individual subjects. It tests the null hypotheses that repeated VOR testing at weekly intervals results in insignificant habituation. It serves as a control for a companion report describing clinical application of the VAT for weekly monitoring of cis-platin vestibulo-toxicity [8].

Methods

Four subjects without histories of vestibular disorders were tested in the light with 3 horizontal and 3 vertical VAT on each of 3 test days. The six tests were conducted at the same time of the day on each of three days separated by weekly intervals, for a total of 9 horizontal and 9 vertical VAT on each subject.

During horizontal VAT, seated subjects were instructed to shake their heads smoothly from side-to-side in the horizontal plane in synchrony with an audible click as a frequency cue. The click frequency increased linearly from 0.5 to 6 Hz during 18 s. The subjects fixated on a 1-cm spot at a known distance from the eyes throughout the test. Tests were separated by 1-min rest periods. Following 3 horizontal VAT, 3 vertical VAT were conducted with the same protocol, but with head and eye motion in a nose up-down, vertical plane.

Horizontal eye movements were recorded by electro-oculography with bilateral electrodes placed at the outer canthi, and a reference electrode above the bridge of the nose. Vertical eye movements were recorded from electrodes placed above and below one eye. Head velocity was recorded with a lightweight, calibrated rotational velocity sensor fixed to an adjustable headband. Eye position and head velocity information were amplified and digitized with IBM-compatible computers equipped with data acquisition peripherals. Eye velocity was computed by a central difference differentiation of eye position, using algorithms described previously [6]. Eye velocity was calibrated from the early, slow head-eye movements by a linear regression fit of eye and (calibrated) head velocities [9]. Gain and phase at frequencies greater than 2 Hz were computed by discrete Fourier analysis, using conventional linear system definitions [6].

Gain and phase data at each frequency were analyzed statistically with the distribution-free Kruskall-Wallis test to determine the ($p < 0.05$) significance of (1) intra-subject weekly differences, and (2) inter-subject grouped differences.

Results

Figure 1 shows eye and head trajectories from one test. Eye position amplitude (fig. 1a) was typically less than 15°, which was less than that necessary to cause nystagmus. Peak head velocity (fig. 1b) typically increased to values between 80 and 200 °/s. Eye velocity (fig. 1c) smoothly followed (reversed polarity) head velocity, but with decreased relative peak amplitude during the final 6 s.

Figure 2a, b shows means and standard deviations (SD) of horizontal gain (a) and phase (b) from nine tests on one subject. The gain SD from this subject was about 0.03, and the phase SD was less than 3° at all frequencies. These variances were the same as those obtained from nine serial tests on another subject, with 3-min rest intervals.

Results of the Kruskall-Wallis test indicated insignificant week-to-week differences among the 9 gain or phase trajectories from this subject and also two others. In the fourth subject, apparent week-to-week differences in both gain and phase at frequencies above 3 Hz were found to be artifacts caused by a looser head strap during one week's test. Tightening the strap resulted in raising the artifactually lowered gains and increased phase lags to within smaller ranges for this subject, and tests of these ranges showed insignificant week-to-week differences for this subject as well.

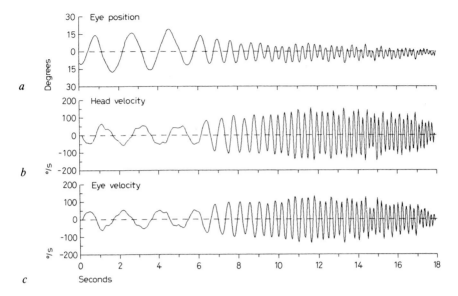

Fig. 1. Horizontal VOR eye and head movement trajectories. *a* Eye position; *b* head velocity; *c* eye velocity.

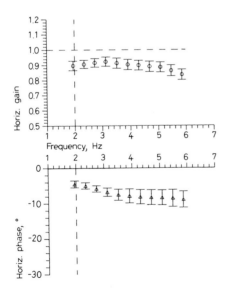

Fig. 2. Horizontal VOR gains from nine repeated VAT tests on the same subject. o, Δ = means; error bars = 1 SD. Three tests were conducted on each of 3 days at weekly intervals.

Differences among subjects' mean gains and phases from all 9 tests were insignificant (Kruskall-Wallis test) [10]. However, the SD of the ensemble data from the 9 tests on all 4 subjects were *greater* than those shown in figure 2 for one subject. The multiple-subject SD in this study agreed with those reported previously from tests on 15 different subjects, each tested once [6].

Discussion

Our results indicate that use of active head movements with sweep frequencies provided a reliable, reproducible method of vestibulo-ocular analysis at higher frequency ranges. The standard deviations of multiple tests on individual subjects were relatively narrow, even when the tests were separated by weekly intervals. Furthermore, week-to-week habituation was not statistically evident. Absence of habituation sugests that this method is useful for weekly diagnostic monitoring for specific clinical disorders [7]. A companion report describes its use in weekly monitoring of cis-platin vestibulo-toxicity [8].

References

1   Gresty, M.A.; Hess, K.; Leech, J.: Disorders of the vestibulo-ocular reflex producing oscillopsia and mechanisms compensating for loss of labyrinthine function. Brain *100:* 693–716 (1977).

2   Istl, Y.E.; Hyden, D.; Schwarz, W.F.: Quantification and localization of vestibular loss in unilaterally labyrinthectomized patients using a precise rotatory test. Acta oto-lar. *96:* 437-445 (1983).

3   Hyden, D.; Larsby, B.; Schwarz, D.W.F.; Odkvist, L.M.: Quantification of slow compensatory eye movements in patients with bilateral vestibular loss. Acta oto-lar. *96:* 11–206 (1983).

4   Hyden, D.; Istl, Y.E.; Schwarz, D.W.F.: Human visuo-vestibular interaction as a basis for quantitative clinical diagnostics. Acta oto-lar. *94:* 53–60 (1982).

5   Tomlinson, R.D.; Saunders, G.E.; Schwarz, D.W.F.: Analysis of human vestibulo-ocular reflex during active head movements. Acta oto-lar. *90:* 184-190 (1980).

6   Fineberg, R.; O'Leary, D.P.; Davis, L.: Use of active head movements for computerized vestibular testing. Archs Otolar. *113:* 1063–1065 (1987).

7   Kitsigianis, G.A.; O'Leary, D.P.; Davis, L.: Active head movement analysis of cis-platin induced vestibulo-toxicity. Otolaryngol. Head Neck Surg. *98:* 82–87 (1988).

8 Kitsigianis, G.A.; O'Leary, D.P.; Davis, L.: Vestibular autorotation testing of cis-platin chemotherapy patients. Adv Oto-Rhino-Laryng., vol. 42, pp. 250–253 (Karger, Basel 1988).

9 Mansson A.; Vesterhauge, S.: A new and simple calibration of the electro-ocular signal for vestibular-ocular measurements. Aviat. Space Envir. Med *58:* suppl. 9, pp. A231–A235 (1987).

10 Hollander, M.; Wolfe, D.A.: Nonparametric statistical methods. (Wiley & Sons, Chichester 1973).

Dennis P. O'Leary, PhD, Vestibular Laboratory, University of Southern California School of Medicine, Parkview Medical Buildings, C-103, 1420 San Pablo Street, Los Angeles, CA 90033 (USA)

Adv. Oto-Rhino-Laryng., vol. 41, pp. 184–189 (Karger, Basel 1988)

Influence of the Vestibular Stimulation on the Activity of Muscles of the Lower Limb in Man. Electromyographic Evidence

S. Marcellini, G.C. Modugno, A. Rinaldi Ceroni, E. Pirodda

Clinica Otorinolaringologica dell' Università di Bologna, Bologna, Italy

The clinical evaluation of the efficiency of vestibulo-spinal reflexes has been and is essentially founded on the subjective observation of the effects on the body posture or on the body movements of the asymmetry in the tonus of skeletal musculature induced by spontaneous or experimentally elicited vestibular imbalance.

Attempts at working out procedures for an objective, quantitative evaluation of the muscular reflex activity and of the reflex gain did not offer conclusive and practically utilizable results. In particular, investigations on changes induced by vestibular stimulation in the EMG [3, 11] did not lead to useful conclusions. In the clinical context, therefore, procedures involvin global measurement of the magnitude of the displacement of the body o the limbs induced by the asymmetry of tonic influences at present hnu increasing diffusion [4, 8, 9]. However, since EMG unquestionably appears to be the most suitable means of investigating muscular activity in its objective qualitative as well as quantitative characteristics, it is worthwhile trying to apply modern procedures of analysis of EMG to the study of the vestibulo-spinal reflexes. This procedure stems from the consideration of the nature and properties of muscular activity and of the multiplicities of afferent stimuli which can influence this activity, thus making it difficult to achieve an isolated evaluation of the influence of the vestibular input.

Mathematical analysis of spectrum power has been found to be a very useful tool in the characterization of myoelectric signals [1]. Shifts in the frequency spectrum have been observed as an expression of different functional situations [2, 5–7, 10]. The mean frequency as well as the median frequency (MF) — 'defined as the frequency value which divides the ME signal power spectrum into two sections of equal energy content' — have been found to provide a good representation of the frequency shift.

Materials and Methods

The present study was carried out on 7 normal healthy young subjects (mean age 28 years). EMG was recorded for a series of constant-force voluntary contractions (CVC) (each of 5 s duration) of the tibialis anterior muscle (dorso-flexion movement of the foot). An appropriate device was utilized to insure the best possible uniformity in the contraction strength and in the flexion angle of the foot. The subject was lying in the supine position, the head bent forward by 30°. Recordings were taken before and after caloric stimulation of the homolateral labyrinth.

The sequence of tests and recordings proceeded as follows: CVC, 5 s; rest, 15 s; CVC, 5 s before the vestibular stimulation. CVC, 5 s; rest, 15 s repeated five times following the vestibular stimulation. On each subject the EMG characteristics of activity recorded during maximal voluntary contraction (MVC) of the same muscle were also determined. Different vestibular stimuli were used on 2 subjects (20, 30, 40, 46 °C), the experimental protocol being slightly modified (the sequence 5 s CVC – 15 s rest was repeated three times before and ten times following the vestibular stimulation). In 2 cases the EMG taken from the gastrocnemius muscle under parallel experimental conditions was also recorded.

The interferential recordings, obtained from surface electrodes placed parallel to the course of muscle fibres (at the proximal third of the muscle) by a Medelec MS6 amplifier were filtered between 32 and 500 Hz, digitized through an A-D converter at 1,000 Hz of sampling rate. Samples corresponding to each 5-second recording were divided into 20 data-blocks of 250 ms. The median frequency was calculated on each data-block, by means of an algorithm of Fast-Fourier Transform, with a 6502 processor. The non-randomness of the behaviour of MF versus time, for each single subject, was checked by using two non-parametric statistic methods (runs test up and down, runs test above and below median). In order to identify the function which best describes this behaviour, the algorithm of non-linear regression by Marquardt was applied.

The difference between MF values obtained in CVC and in the MVC was submitted to statistical evaluation by the Kolmogorov-Smirnov two-sample test.

Results

In all of the tested subjects MF of EMG recorded from the tibialis anterior muscle showed, in comparison to the basal values, increased values following the warm vestibular stimulation (H_2O 44 °C).

MF was back to pre-stimulatory values within 2–3 min. Such behaviour cannot be considered a random occurrence. The interpolation curve which best represents it, is a third-order curve (fig. 1).

In all of the tested subjects MF values corresponding to the MVC were significantly higher ($p < 0.01$) than values obtained during CVC, both before and following the vestibular stimulation (table I).

The cold caloric stimulation (H_2O 30 °C) induced a decrease in the values of MF, in comparison with pre-stimulatory values, which was followed

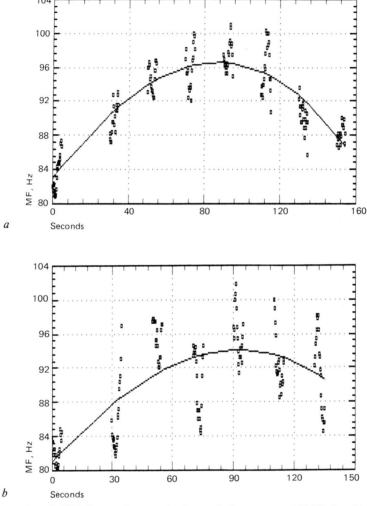

Fig. 1. Tibialis anterior muscle: interpolation curves of EMG data-blocks from 2 subjects.

by a gradual return to initial basal values within 3–5 min (fig. 2). When stimuli of different magnitude were used, the increase or decrease in the MF values were found to be proportionally related to the intensity of stimulation (fig. 2).

Values of MF in the EMG taken from the gastrocnemius muscle showed a specular behaviour with respect to those corresponding to the tibialis anterior muscle when a warm stimulation was performed (fig. 3). No

Table I. Median frequencies during an isometric voluntary constant-force contraction (CVC) and during a maximal voluntary contraction (MVC) — median value

Subjects	CVC[1]	MVC[1]	Var., %	Significance level*
1	91	118	29.67	< 0.01
2	76	93	22.37	< 0.01
3	140	171	22.14	< 0.01
4	83	105	26.51	< 0.01
5	125	160	28.00	< 0.01
6	80	94	17.50	< 0.01
7	85	113	32.94	< 0.01

[1] Sign test for location.
*Kolmogorov-Smirnov two-sample test.

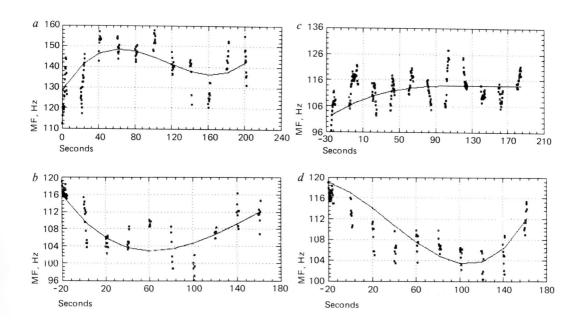

Fig. 2. Tibialis anterior muscle: interpolation curves of EMG data-blocks corresponding to different magnitudes of vestibular stimuli. *a* H_2O 46 °C; *b* H_2O 40 °C; *c* H_2O 30 °C; *d* H_2O 20 °C.

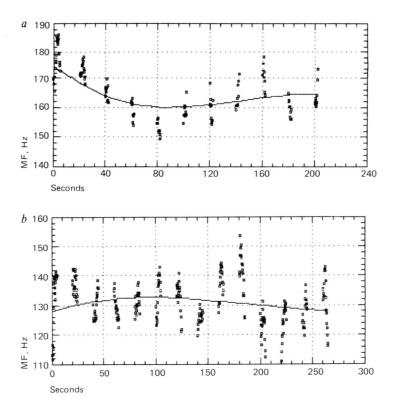

Fig. 3. Gastrocnemius muscle: interpolation curves of EMG data-blocks corresponding to: *a* warm vestibular stimulation; *b* cold vestibular stimulation.

significant (constant) results were obtained in the few cases where a cold
stimulation was applied (fig. 3).

Discussion and Conclusions

The results we have described seem to prove convincingly that changes
in the electrical activity of inferior limb muscles induced by vestibular
stimulation can be reliably and constantly recorded and analyzed under
clinical conditions.

All of the tested subjects showed a shift in the values of the MF of the
power spectrum of EMG, the pattern of which satisfactorily paralleled the
course of events elicited by the applied vestibular (caloric) stimulation.

In our opinion, such a finding is sufficient to motivate a more extended and systematic study of the behaviour of the electrical activity of skeletal muscles under the influence of different vestibular stimuli. A complete set of observations could provide useful data for a fruitful comparison with electrophysiological findings in animals. The results of our experiments, on the other hand, indicate that an objective demonstration and possibly a quantitative evaluation of the vestibulo-spinal reflex activity of skeletal muscles becomes possible.

Complexities in the processes of analysis, even in the light of presently available computing possibilities, can be relatively easily overcome.

References

1 Basmajian, J.V.; De Luca, C.J.: Muscles alive (Williams & Wilkins, Baltimore 1985).
2 Broman, H.; Bilotto, G.; De Luca, C.J.: Myoelectric signal conduction velocity and spectral parameters: influence of force and time. J. appl. Physiol. 58: 1428–1437 (1985).
3 Emami-Nuori, M.: Eine elektromyographische Studie über die vestibularen Reflexe. Lar. Rhinol. 54: 512–530 (1975).
4 Igarashi, M.; Black, P.O.: Vestibular and visual control on posture and locomotor equilibrium (Karger, Basel 1985).
5 Kranz, H.; Williams, A.M.; Cassell, J.; Caddy, D.J.; Silberstein, R.B.: Factors determining the frequency content of the electromyogram. J. appl. Physiol. 55: 392–399 (1983).
6 Marletti, R.; Sabbahi, M.A.; De Luca, C.J.: Median frequency of the myoelectric signal. Effects of muscle ischemia and cooling. Eur. J. appl. Physiol. 52: 258–265 (1984).
7 Merletti, R.; Castagno, F.; Prato, G.; Saracco, C.; Pisani, R.: Proprietá e ripetibilitá di misura di parametri spettrali del segnale EMG cutaneo in soggetti normali. Rass. Bioing. 10: 83–96 (1985).
8 Nashner, L.: The organization of human postural movements: a formal basis and experimental synthesis. Behav. Brain Sci. 8: 135–172 (1985).
9 Norre, M.E.: La posturographie en otoneurologie. Cah. ORL 19: 15–23 (1985).
10 Sabbahi. M.A.; Merletti, R.; De Luca, C.J.; Rosenthal, R.G.: How handiness, sex and force level affect the median frequency of the myoelectric signal; in Trimble, Doubler, Heckathorne, Proc. 4th Annu. Conf. on Rehabilitation Engineering, Washington 1981.
11 Strobel, H.: Elektromyographische Untersuchungen über den Einfluss des Vestibularapparates auf die tonische Aktivität der quergestreiften Muskulatur beim Menschen. Arch. klin. exp. Ohr.- Nas.-Kehlk. Heilk. 198: 187–205 (1971).

S. Marcellini, MD, Clinica Otorinolaringologica dell'Universitá di Bologna,
Via Massarenti 9, I-40138 Bologna (Italy)

Adv. Oto-Rhino-Laryng., vol. 41, pp. 190–195 (Karger, Basel 1988)

Test-Retest Reliability of the Rotatory Test in Normal Subjects

Herman A. Jenkins, Jefim Goldberg[1]

Clayton Foundation for Research Neurotology Laboratory,
Department of Otorhinolaryngology and Communicative Sciences,
Baylor College of Medicine, Houston, Tex., USA

Introduction

Documentation of changes in vestibulo-ocular responses induced by vestibular and organ disease remains a difficult task due to the high variability in patients' responses to vestibular stimulation. This is particularly true in quantification of disease progression. The caloric test, while providing a means of assessment of individual ear function, is too imprecise to adequately measure subtle variations in vestibulo-ocular reflex parameters in chronic labyrinthine disease [1–3]. The rotatory test offers a means of quantitative evaluation of vestibular function using precisely controlled, computer-assisted stimulation. It has been advocated as a tool to monitor progressive changes in vestibular function in a variety of situations. The present study was undertaken to evaluate this potential. A series of experiments was designed to determine the reproducibility of results obtained with rotatory testing within individual subjects tested on multiple occasions.

Materials and Methods

Twelve normal healthy subjects without any history of auditory or vestibular dysfunction were used in the study. Subjects ranged in age from 22 to 27 with a mean of 24.1 ± 2.3 years and included 6 men and 6 women. Each subject was tested on six separate

[1] The authors wish to acknowledge Dr. Paul Swank for his contributions to the statistical analysis, Margaret Kallsen for programming and Elisa Icaza and Dr. Eric Furst for technical assistance.

occasions one week apart. Care was taken to adhere to a strict protocol, with testing sessions being performed on the same day of the week and at the same hour of the day to rule out, as much as possible, extraneous effects, e.g. diurnal variation.

During an experimental session the subject was seated in a servo-controlled rotatory chair (Contraves-Goertz) inside a dark, sound-dampened room. Eye position was recorded using DC-coupled electro-oculography with calibrations performed before and after each rotation. Chair rotation was controlled by a DEC LSI 11/23 minicomputer which also digitized eye position and chair velocity signals. In each session, the subject was rotated in the dark at seven sinusoidal frequencies ranging from 0.00625 to 0.4 Hz with peak velocities of 60°/s. During testing subjects were instructed to keep their eyes open as if looking straight ahead and to perform mental alerting tasks. Eye movement data were analyzed using an iterative technique of progressive smoothing of the data to remove fast phase activity and the resultant data curve-fitted to obtain measures of gain, phase, asymmetry and DC bias. Testing conditions and analysis have been reported elsewhere in greater detail [4].

Results

The vestibulo-ocular reflex responses induced by sinusoidal rotation can be described by four parameters: gain, phase, asymmetry and DC bias. These quantities were determined for each of the six repetitions of the rotatory test for the individual subjects. Based on these data, figures 1 and 2 illustrate the consistency of the vestibulo-ocular reflex parameter measurements across repetitions. The measurements plotted against frequency of rotation for one subject are shown in figure 1. The shaded areas indicate the ranges of parameter values obtained in the six repetitions, while the dots and bars represent the means and standard deviations of these values.

Of the four parameters, phase values (upper right) showed the best reproducibility. At all frequencies, variability of this parameter was low, with the standard deviation being no greater than 3° at any frequency. The variabilities of gain and DC bias were greater; gain standard deviation varied from 17% of the mean at the lowest frequency to 7% for the highest. Asymmetry showed the greatest variability.

Figure 2 summarizes the within-subject variability of vestibulo-ocular reflex measurements in the test population of 12 normal subjects. For each parameter the shaded area represents the range of measurement standard deviations found in the population, while the dots and bars represent the mean and standard deviation of these values. As can be seen (fig. 2), the within-subject standard deviations vary considerably between individuals and between test frequencies.

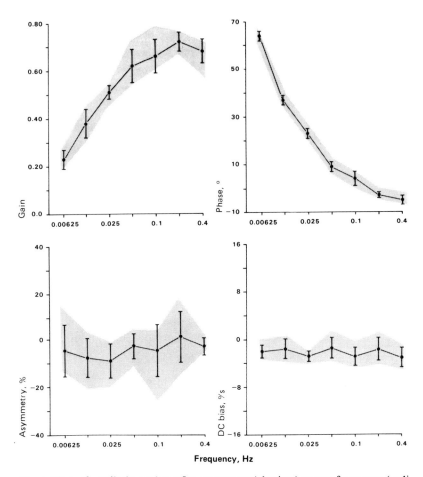

Fig. 1. Plots of vestibulo-ocular reflex parameter (abscissa) versus frequency (ordinate). Shaded area indicates range of values, dot and bars represent the mean and standard deviation of the six repetitions.

Generalizability analysis [5] was used to determine the reliability coefficients for each of the calculated parameters (see Discussion). Figure 3 illustrates the reliability coefficients of these parameters, calculated for observations made on one (triangles), three (squares) and six (circles) occasions for the seven test frequencies. As would be predicted, all parameters showed their highest reliability when tested on six occasions. In generalizability analysis coefficients range from zero to one with zero corresponding to no reliability (all error) and one to perfect reliability (no error). For scientific purposes coefficients above 0.7 are considered adequate. Gain measures

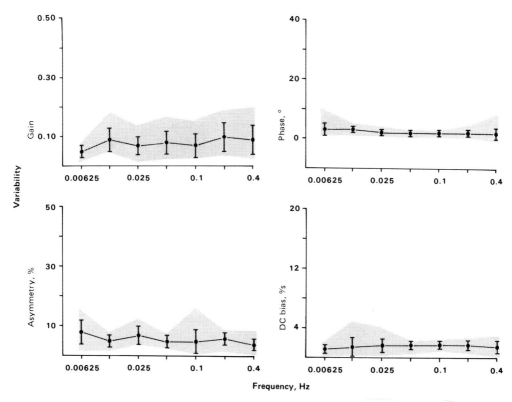

Fig. 2. Plots of the intersubject variability of the vestibulo-ocular reflex parameters versus frequency. The shaded area indicates the range for the standard deviations of the six repetitions in the individual subjects and the dots and bars the mean and standard deviations of these values.

obtained from testing on three or six occasions showed reliability greater than 0.7 across all frequencies. When tested on one occasion, the lowest and three midfrequency tests showed acceptable reliability.

Phase similarly showed excellent reliability across all frequencies when tested on three and six occasions. However, when tested on only one occasion reliability was only acceptable for frequencies below 0.2 Hz. Asymmetry showed adequate reliability coefficients only when tested on six occasions at the midfrequencies of 0.025 and 0.05 Hz. Reliability of this parameter fell off dramatically both at the higher frequencies and when tested on fewer occasions. DC bias measurements were sufficiently reliable when tested on

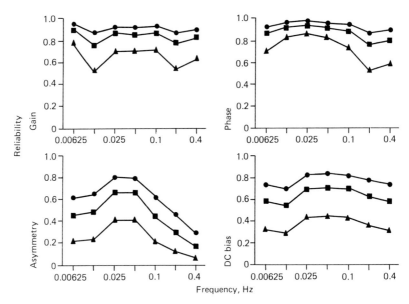

Fig. 3. Reliability coefficients for each of the parameters versus frequency. Triangles represent coefficients for one, squares three and circles six repetitions.

six occasions and on three for the midfrequency range 0.025 to 0.1 Hz. For testing on one occasion, reliability was very low.

Discussion

A measurement must have two properties to be acceptable: validity and reliability. Validity is the degree to which a measure assesses the trait in question, i.e. the accuracy. Reliability is the degree to which the measurements are consistent, i.e. reproducible from one trial to another. Good test reliability is necessary so that differences in vestibulo-ocular reflex responses between individuals will not be obscured by variability of the measurements within individuals.

Generalizability analysis was used to estimate the contributions of (repeated) measurement variability versus interindividual differences to variation in vestibulo-ocular response measurements in a narrowly defined population of healthy subjects. The generalizability coefficient for a single replicate reflects the proportion of variance in the observations for a single occasion which is due to actual differences between individuals. For multiple replicates, the coefficient reflects the proportion of variance in the means of the multiple observations which is due to actual mean differences between individuals.

In this study the resulting reliability coefficients were acceptable for a single measurement of the gain parameter at frequencies of 0.00625, 0.025, 0.05 and 0.1 Hz. For a single phase measurement reliability was acceptable at frequencies below 0.2 Hz. Asymmetry and DC bias were not sufficiently reliable at any frequency.

These results can be considered a 'worst case' analysis since our population was chosen to minimize interindividual differences. In practice, the relative reliability should be higher when the test population includes a wider age distribution as well as patients with vestibular deficits. Repeating a test will always increase its reliability. The present analysis was confined to a single rotatory frequency at a time. Since vestibulo-ocular reflex tests are typically performed at several frequencies, proper combination of these test results should improve reliability, just as repeating the test does.

This study permits some conclusions to be drawn as to which is the best or most reliable frequency for patient testing. Subjecting patients to a wide range of frequencies is often not possible due to time constraints and the physical condition of the patient. Inclusion of midfrequencies in the testing paradigm would offer the best reliability, particularly when testing at only a single or few frequencies is to be performed on only a single occasion.

References

1   Coats, A.C; Hebert. F.; Atwood, G.R.: The air caloric test. Archs Otolar. *102:* 343–357 (1976).
2   Proctor, L.; Glackin, R.: Factors contributing to variability of caloric test scores. Acta oto-lar. *100:* 161–171 (1985).
3   Honrubia, V.; Jenkins, H.A.; Minser, K.; Baloh, R.W.; Yee, R.D.: Vestibulo-ocular reflexes in peripheral labyrinthine lesions. II. Caloric testing. Am. J. Otolaryngol. *5:* 93–98 (1984).
4   Jenkins, H.A.: Long-term adaptive changes of the vestibulo-ocular reflex in patients following acoustic neuroma surgery. Laryngoscope *95:* 1224–1234 (1985).
5   Cronbach, L.J.; Glesar, G.C.; Nanda, H.; Rajaratnam, N.: The dependability of behavioral measurements. Theory of generalizability for scores and profiles (Wiley, New York 1972).

Herman A. Jenkins, MD, Clayton Foundation for Research Neurotology Laboratory, Department of Otorhinolaryngology and Communicative Sciences, Baylor College of Medicine, Houston, TX 77030 (USA)

Adv. Oto-Rhino-Laryng., vol. 41, pp. 196–200 (Karger, Basel 1988)

Beat-to-Beat Variability of Nystagmus.
A Clinical Study

Ilmari Pyykkö[a], *Martti Juhola*[b]

[a]Department of Otolaryngology, University Hospital of Helsinki, Helsinki;
[b]Department of Computer Science, University of Turku, Turku, Finland

Introduction

In the rotatory test different patterns of nystagmus have been observed that may be indicative for dysrhythmia of nystagmus [Pyykkö et al., 1984; Pyykkö and Dahlen, 1985a, b]. Honrubia et al. [1980] described prominent amplitude variations of nystagmus which could be connected with the site of the lesion. According to these authors, in the presence of a central vestibular lesion the nystagmus will be disorganized and the fast components occur in random fashion, especially when the lesion involves the cerebellum. In only a few reports, however, has dysrhythmia of nystagmus been analysed quantitatively.

The purpose of the present study was to evaluate the sequential variability of nystagmus in three groups of patients. The results indicate that in patients with a frontal lobe lesion and in patients with a brain stem lesion there is a significant change in the processing of nystagmus, indicating ailment of the brain circuitries controlling the velocity, time and amplitude of nystagmus.

Subjects

Ten normal subjects, aged 25–62 years, were recruited for the determination of normative values [Pyykkö et al., 1987]. Thirty patients with different neurological diseases were selected for this study: (Group 1) 10 patients with acute vestibular neuronitis; (Group 2) 10 patients with frontal lobe lesion; (Group 3) 10 patients with brain stem lesion.

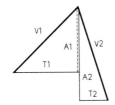

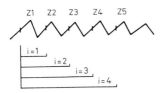

Fig, 1, Variables of nystagmus beat. $V1$ = Slow phase velocity; $V2$ = fast phase velocity; $T1$ = slow phase duration; $T2$ = fast phase duration; $A1$ = slow phase amplitude; $A2$ = fast phase amplitude.

Methods

The horizontal eye movements were recorded binocularly and the vertical eye movements from each eye separately. The positional signal of the eyes was recorded with an ink-jet recorder (Mingograph M82, Siemens Elema, Stockholm, Sweden). An upper cut-off frequency of 15 Hz with infinite time constant was used.

The subjects were exposed to the Bárány rotatory test. The chair was accelerated in dark with eyes open within 1 s to a speed of 120 °/s. The rotation lasted 60 s, after which the chair was decelerated to a standstill within 1 s. The analysis was limited to postrotatory response.

To analyse the sequential variability between different components (fig. 1) within the nystagmus response, the data were fed into a minicomputer (PDP-11-23, Digital Equipment). Interactive programs were developed by which linear regression analysis between different qualities of nystagmus could be performed. In the program a comparison between the y- and x-axis was made by relating continuously selected components of two beats together, i.e. $Z1$, with $Z1+i$, $Z2$ with $Z2+i$, $Z3$ with $Z3+i$, etc. where i was 1. The difference between the various groups of patients was analysed with analysis of variance. The difference was statistically significant when p was less than 0.05.

Results

In the slow phase velocity ($V1$) all patients had a significant correlation with successive $V1$. The correlation coefficients and standard error for regression for patients with frontal lobe lesions was 0.680 (Sr = 13.09), for brain stem lesions 0.767 (Sr = 8.93), for vestibular end organ lesion 0.847 (Sr = 8.69) and for normal controls 0.880 (Sr = 8.10). The patients with frontal lobe lesion had significantly lower correlation coefficients (p <0.001) and larger standard errors for regression (p <0.01) than other groups of subjects.

In the interbeat relationship between successive slow phase amplitudes (A1) all groups of patients had a significant correlation in their nystagmus responses. The correlation coefficients and standard error for regression (Sr) were 0.273 (Sr = 5.56) for the frontal lobe patients, 0.434 (Sr = 3.67) for the brain stem patients, 0.355 (Sr = 4.19) for the peripheral vestibular lesion patients and 0.3466 (Sr = 3.81) for normal controls. The patients with frontal lobe lesion had significantly lower correlation coefficient (p <0.05) and higher intercept (p <0.05) than other groups. It is noteworthy that the patients with brain stem lesion show remarkably high correlation coefficients but also have a significantly low intercept (p <0.001) when compared with other groups of patients.

In the duration of nystagmus (T1) the patients with brain stem lesions (r = 0.276, SR = 0.06) and with frontal lobe lesions (r = 0.227, Sr = 0.14) differed significantly from the patients with vestibular end organ lesion (r = 0.403, Sr = 0.09) and normal controls (r = 0.433, Sr = 0.05) in both having lower correlation (p <0.05) and higher standard error of regression (p <0.01). Thus, nystagmus duration varied significantly in brain stem patients and frontal lobe patients when compared to normal subjects.

In fast phase components of nystagmus no significant differences were observed between any of the groups and normal subjects.

Discussion

Attempts to study the relationship between the different variables of nystagmus have only recently been made. Buizza et al. [1978] and Schmid [1982] have employed the ratio between the duration of each pair of successive nystagmus beats and the ratio between the amplitudes of each pair of successive fast components. One or both of the so-called interbeat relationships could be pathological and, therefore, characterize the underlying lesion in the vestibular system. So far, clinical applications of this method have been limited to case reports. In the present study with respect to dysrhythmia in slow phase velocity only patients with frontal lobe showed larger beat-to-beat variability whereas in other groups no such variability was observed. In duration of slow phase dysrhythmia was significant in patients with a brain stem and with a frontal lobe lesion.

We did not find that fast phase velocity, amplitude or duration would be the major source of dysrhythmia. The lack of any apparent correlation in the fast phase of nystagmus in the sequential model indicates that the variations of nystagmus qualities linked to the fast phase in control subjects and in patients are normally vast in postrotatory nystagmus. Consequently, the dysrhythmias in the fast phase may not be as useful as had been proposed earlier [Buizza et al., 1978].

Short periods of absence of nystagmus have been considered to be due to an abrupt change in nystagmus velocity and are indicative of a central vestibular lesion (Fluur, 1982]. In the present study nystagmus velocity variations were found during the postrotatory responses in greater extent than normally among patients with a frontal lobe lesion. The improper nystagmus response among the frontal lobe patients may be derived from a lesion in the frontal eye field that controls the execution of nystagmus [cf. Hoyt and Frisen, 1975].

Fluur and Mendel [1963] explained that dysrhythmia is a normal phenomenon and linked to adaptive vestibular responses. Since the pathological signs of dysrhythmia in the present study were mainly linked to slow phase velocity, it is reasonable to assume that the majority of deviations, either in time or amplitude frame of nystagmus, are normal findings. The present model does not include all possibilities of dysrhythmia, i.e. temporary beat-to-beat variations. Therefore, other methods to analyse such variations should be researched. As shown in another study, intrabeat analysis of dysrhythmia provides important information on the variation of the end point of nystagmus [Pyykkö and Dahlen, 1985b].

References

Buizza, A.; Schmid, R.; Zanibelli, A.; Mira, E.; Semplici, P.: Quantification of vestibular nystagmus by an interactive computer program. ORL *40:* 147 (1978).

Fluur, E.: Clinical investigation of the efferent inhibition of the vestibular function. Acta oto-lar. *94:* 495 (1982).

Honrubia, V.; Baloh, R.W.; Yee, R.D.; Jenkins, H.A.: Identification of the location of vestibular lesions on the basis of vestibulo-ocular reflex measurements. Am. J. Otolaryngol. *1:* 291 (1980).

Hoyt, W.F.; Frisen, L.: Supranuclear ocular motor control. Some clinical considerations; in Lennerstrand, Bach-y-Rita, Basic mechanisms of ocular motility and their clinical implications, pp. 379–394 (Pergamon Press, Oxford 1975).

Pyykkö, I.; Dahlen, A.-I.: Intrabeat relationship of postrotatory nystagmus in normal subjects. Acta oto-lar. *99:* 74–82 (1985a).

Pyykkö, I.; Dahlen, A.-I.: Intrabeat relationship of postrotatory nystagmus in patients with neurological disorders. Acta oto-lar. *99:* 113–121 (1985b).

Pyykkö, I.; Dahlen, A.-I.; Henriksson, N.G.; Juhola, M.: Clinical evaluation of dysrhythmia of postrotatory nystagmus. Acta oto-lar. *98:* 279–286 (1984).

Pyykkö, I.; Juhola, M.; Henriksson, N.G.: Sequential variability of postrotatory nystagmus in normal subjects; in Graham, Kemink, The vestibular system: neurophysiological and clinical research, pp. 341–350 (Raven Press, New York 1987).

Schmid, R.: Technical problems in stimulation, recording, and analysis of eye movements; in Honrubia, Brazier, Nystagmus and vertigo, pp. 81–94 (Academic Press, New York 1982).

Ilmari Pyykkö, MD, Department of Otolaryngology, University Hospital of Helsinki, Haartmaninkatu 2-4 E, SF-00290 Helsinki (Finland)

Adv. Oto-Rhino-Laryng., vol. 41, pp. 201–205 (Karger, Basel 1988)

Comparison of Caloric and OKAN Tests in Patients with Vestibular Deficits

R.M. Jell, H.D. Phillips, S.H. Lafortune, D.J. Ireland

Departments of Physiology and Otolaryngology, University of Manitoba, Winnipeg, Canada

Introduction

Caloric testing has been widely used as a method of assessment of vestibular function in the clinical laboratory; however, the method is far from perfect. Optokinetic afternystagmus (OKAN) is dependent upon semicircular canal [Cohen et al., 1973], central visual and vestibular pathways, as well as upon sensory integrative centres in the brain stem which are responsible for velocity storage [Cohen et al., 1977; Raphan et al., 1979]. Hence, the phenomenon offers the possibility of testing several different aspects of the visual-vestibular system in one test. Rotational tests lack sensitivity in unilateral labyrinthine disease [Honrubia et al., 1982; Tomlinson et al., 1984] and are mainly useful in identifying bilateral labyrinthine deficits [Yee et al., 1978]. In the light of the various difficulties in obtaining accurate clinical data about end organ and/or central integrity, we have been examining the potential usefulness of OKAN testing in an attempt to improve the diagnosis of vestibular disorders. To establish the usefulness of the OKAN test we have compared data obtained from caloric and rotatory testing with results from OKAN testing in 11 chronic vestibular patients.

Methods

Rotational Testing. Patients were subjected to 6 °/s² acceleration for 15 s followed by constant velocity rotation for 60 s and a deceleration of 90 °/s² for 1 s in both clockwise (C) and counterclockwise (CW) directions. The post-rotatory nystagmus (PRN) decay was fitted with a single exponential by linear regression. Decay time constants below 8.5 s were considered to be abnormal.

Table I. Caloric and PRN test results

Patient	Age	Sex	Onset	Caloric deficit	PRN	Diagnosis
M.S.	49	M	July 82	NCD	N	post trauma
H.H.	32	M	Mar. 85	NCD	—	BPPN
C.D.	32	F	Sept. 84	NCD	N	normal
K.H.	45	M	Jan. 83	NCD	N	post trauma
E.B.	27	F	? 77	NCD	A	Ménière's
A.G.	74	M	Jan. 85	LT 38%	N	vestib. neuronitis
H.G.	52	F	Aug. 84	LT 43%	N	post trauma
B.K.	25	M	Sept. 84	LT 43%	N	?
M.M.	67	F	Aug. 75	RT 33%	N	vestib. neuronitis
J.B.	55	F	Aug. 82	RT 35%	N	vestib. neuronitis
J.G.	47	F	Apr. 83	RT 100%	A	vestib. neuronitis

NCD = No caloric deficit; N = normal; A = abnormal PRN.

Caloric Testing. Standard bithermal Hallpike caloric tests were performed at 44 and 30 °C for a period of 30 s. Eye movements were recorded by standard EOG. The SPV points were digitized at the peak of the response (10 s of data). Jongkees' formula was used to determine the reduced vestibular response with normal limits being ± 22%.

OKAN Testing. Patients were exposed to 60 s of constant velocity (40 °/s) optokinetic (OK) stimulation (in both C and CW directions) by means of an OK drum consisting of a white curtain lined with black vertical stripes (2° wide) at 18° intervals. Distance of eyes to the drum was 33 cm. OKAN decay was recorded for 60 s after lights out, and fitted by non-linear regression to the double exponential equation of the form: $SPV = A \exp(-Bt) + C \exp(-Dt)$ [Jell et al., 1984]. A and C are the coefficients of the short time constant (1/B) and long time constant (1/D) components, respectively. The coefficients and time constants as well as the integral of the slow phase velocities (i.e. area under the decay curve which is an estimate of total eye displacement) were used as OKAN measurement parameters.

Results

Results from caloric and PRN testing, and relevant information about the patients, are presented in table I. The OKAN measurement parameters obtained (coefficients, time constants and area under the decay) are shown in table II. Most of the values for coefficient C and long time constant 1/D were found to be outside the normal range. The values which indicate the sidedness of the disorder appear in italics.

Table II. OKAN decay parameters. Values indicating the side of the lesion are italicized

Patient	Caloric deficit	A	1/B	C	1/D	Total area	Diagnosis
M.S.	NCD	dl 51.0	0.2*	10.9	18.0*	157.7	post trauma
		dr 20.2	0.5	9.8	14.6*	165.8	
H.H.	NCD	27.1	0.8	6.9	16.8*	127.2	BPPN
		35.0	0.7	3.2*	945.5*	211.3	
C.D.	NCD	12.8	0.9	11.3	47.4	397.4	normal
		38.3	2.0	5.0*	38.5	186.0	
K.H.	NCD	50.8	0.3*	6.2	*89.8**	292.5	post trauma
		8.5	1.2	6.4	26.8	158.6	
E.B.	NCD	39.9	0.7	*0.0**	*0.0**	36.9	Ménière's
		50.0	0.5	*0.0**	*0.0**	62.4	(bilateral)
A.G.	LT 38%	19.6	0.5	3.9*	12.2*	63.4	vestib.
		26.4	0.5	*1.1**	19.9*	*34.5*	neuronitis
H.G.	LT 43%	31.1	0.7	1.7*	37.1	63.2	post trauma
		34.2	0.7	*0.0**	*0.0**	*33.8*	
B.K.	LT 43%	18.5	1.0	7.7	10.3*	84.1	?
		18.2	*5.8**	*0.0**	*0.0**	120.1	
M.M.	RT 33%	34.2	1.0	*4.0**	*15.0**	*70.0*	vestib.
		7.7	1.9	6.9	24.1	98.5	neuronitis
J.B.	RT 35%	28.4	0.7	10.8	*4.7**	*67.7*	vestib.
		44.6	0.8	6.8	35.4	171.8	neuronitis
J.G.	RT 100%	43.0	*0.3**	*1.2**	*24.3*	*21.0*	vestib.
		15.9	0.7	8.3	717.5*	546.7	neuronitis
Means	(of 14	35.1	1.2	10.8	48.8	—	—
SD	normals)	29.1	0.8	5.0	26.7		

dl = Drum left (right beating); dr = Drum right (left beating).
* Outside normal limits.

Discussion

The lateralizing value of the OKAN test in unilateral vestibular disease has previously been demonstrated [Ireland and Jell, 1982; Tomlinson et al., 1984]. This lateralizing capability was further confirmed in the present study. In 7 of 11 patients, the side of the lesion or the presence of a bilateral lesion correlated with OKAN measurement parameters (C, 1/D and total area under SPV points). The asymmetry corresponded with that determined by caloric testing. While no caloric deficit could be found in the remaining 4 patients, the OKAN test did reveal some abnormalities, mainly in the long time constant 1/D, the significance of which remains to be determined. However, in these cases, almost all A, 1/B and C values as well as the total areas obtained fell, like the caloric result, within the expected normal range (total area values considered normal lie between 100 and 400°).

The OKAN test can also be used to distinguish central vestibular disorders or brain stem pathology from peripheral loss in the presence of a caloric response [Ireland and Jell, 1984], as in the case of 2 of the present post trauma patients. Deficits revealed by OKAN may be the result of lesions in one or more of many structures (VN, end organs, brain stem, etc.) and more extensive screening of patients and refinement of the OKAN test will be required to clarify this.

In conclusion, the OKAN test can be a valuable clinical tool for revealing peripheral vestibular deficits and sidedness of these deficits.

References

Cohen, B.; Uemura, T.; Takemori, S.: Effects of labyrinthectomy on optokinetic nystagmus (OKN) and optokinetic after-nystagmus (OKAN). Equilib. Res. 3: 88 (1973).
Cohen, B.; Matsuo, V.; Raphan, T.: Quantitative analysis of the velocity characteristics of optokinetic nystagmus and optokinetic after-nystagmus. J. Physiol. 270: 321 (1977).
Honrubia, V.; Jenkins, H.A.; Baloh, R.W.; Lau, C.G.Y.: Evaluation of rotatory vestibular tests in peripheral labyrinthine lesions; in Honrubia, Brazier, Nystagmus and vertigo (Academic Press, New York 1982).
Ireland, D.J.; Jell, R.M.: Optokinetic after-nystagmus in man after loss or reduction of labyrinthine function – a preliminary report. J. Otolaryngol. 11: 86 (1982).
Ireland, D.J.; Jell, R.M.: Symmetrical optokinetic after-nystagmus loss in Wallenberg's syndrome and multiple sclerosis. Acta oto-lar. suppl. 406, p. 235 (1984).
Jell, R.M.; Ireland, D.J.; LaFortune, S.: Human optokinetic afternystagmus. Slow-phase characteristics and analysis of the decay of slow-phase velocity. Acta oto-lar. 98: 462 (1984).

Raphan T.; Matsuo, V.; Cohen B.: Velocity storage in the vestibulo-ocular reflex arc (VOR). Exp. Brain Res. *35:* 229 (1979).

Tomlinson, R.D.; Rubin, A.M.; Wallace, I.R.; Barber H.O.: Optokinetic afternystagmus and post rotatory nystagmus in patients with unilateral labyrinthine lesions. J. Otolaryngol. *13:* 217 (1984).

Yee, R.D.; Jenkins, H.A.; Baloh, R.W.; Honrubia, V.; Lau, C.G.Y.: Vestibular-optokinetic interactions in normal subjects and in patients with peripheral vestibular dysfunction. J. Otolaryngol. *7:* 310 (1978).

R.M. Jell, MD, Departments of Physiology and Otolaryngology,
University of Manitoba, Winnipeg R3E OW3 (Canada)

Adv. Oto-Rhino-Laryng., vol. 41, pp. 206–209 (Karger, Basel 1988)

Rotatory Evoked Potentials in Normal and Labyrinthectomized Rabbits

B. Hofferberth, B. Zünkeler, T. Deitmer, M. Hirschberg

Department of Neurology, University of Münster, Münster, FRG

Introduction

In the past 20 years several investigators have tried to disentangle pure vestibular cortical responses from artifact using galvanic, peri- and postrotatory stimulation while employing increasingly sophisticated data analysis.

Whereas the studies of Kornhuber et al. [1964] and Ödquist et al. [1975] on the cortex of cat and rabbit have provided satisfactory evidence for the vestibular cortex to be located in area 2v and 3a, no consensus can be found as yet concerning the existence and parameters of rotatory evoked vestibular potentials (REP). Latencies of such potentials have shown a puzzling variability among investigators with values ranging from 80 to 500 ms.

In an attempt to clarify whether the REP represented a reproducible means which could be used clinically to detect and differentiate central vestibular defects, we previously examined 30 healthy volunteers and two labyrinthectomized adults [Hofferberth, 1984]. We employed rotational stimuli of considerably lower angular acceleration ($2.5-10°/s^2$) than those commonly used and found characteristic slow potentials with a limited inter- and intra-individual variability and entirely absent response in the two labyrinthectomized patients. However, the question still remained unanswered as to whether the mysterious slow potentials were truly of vestibular origin or, alternatively, were adulterated by other afferences from the somato-periphery. Critics said that the vestibular system, which is a long polysynaptic pathway, including the arousal system of the reticular formation and the medial thalamus, provided plenty of opportunity for such signals to enter.

In order to differentiate between vestibular and other potentials, we decided to do a comparative study with albino rabbits prior to and after labyrinthectomy. The idea was that a REP recording following complete destruction of the labyrinth would enable us to isolate any potentially present overlying signal of primarily non-labyrinthine origin. The advantages of this animal model are a remarkable similarity between the normal REP in rabbits and in humans, the fact that their vestibular-cortical anatomy is known [Ödquist et al., 1975] and the rabbit's somewhat passive psychomotor attitude which proves helpful with respect to artifact suppression.

Material and Methods

In 12 normal, alert albino rabbits the surface EEG was registered using Ag/AgCl electrodes at the occiput versus the nasion, following angular deacceleration stimuli. A computer-controlled motor-driven frame which held the animal firmly inside a rotating dark drum applied the stimuli. Three different angular accelerations were applied sequentially (2.5; 5.0; 7.5 °/s²), each of these in a clockwise and counterclockwise fashion.

The signal thus obtained was processed by a microcomputer (Cromemco CS-1, Z-80) using an 8-bit A/D converter. The sample rate was 1,000/s and 64 sweeps, each following a deacceleration stimulus, were recorded to produce an averaged potential of 500 ms duration. Termination of rotation of the device was used as a trigger. The EEG, EOG, EKG and the chair acceleration were separately and simultaneously documented on a six-channel electroencephalograph (Siemens Mingograph).

In a second experimental step the same animals underwent microsurgical exploration of their middle ears. Coming through the bony auditory meatus, the ossicle chain was luxated and the labyrinth was destroyed by controlled suction through the oval window. Intraoperatively a rapid horizontal nystagmus away from the side of the lesion served as an indicator for successful destruction of the inner ear. To avoid central effects of the short-acting anesthetic agents used, we waited 12 h before REP were taken again.

Results

As shown in figure 1, we found oligophasic REP responses demonstrating four to six peaks of remarkably constant latencies in normal rabbits whereas the peaks in labyrinthectomized animals, if they could be identified at all, showed a much higher variability in their latencies. Median latencies for the most prominent peaks (P2–P4) were: P2, 71.2 ms (SD 8.7 ms); P3, 131.6 ms (SD 18.2 ms); P4, 227.5 ms (SD 24.6 ms) in normal animals. In labyrinthectomized animals only two peaks (P1 and P2) could be identified with any certainty. Median latency for P2 was 88.0 ms (SD 16.5 ms). In normal animals the median peak-to-peak amplitudes were: P2–P3, 9.0 μV (SD 4.8 μV); P3–P4, 13.0 μV (SD 5.1 μV); postoperatively those amplitudes

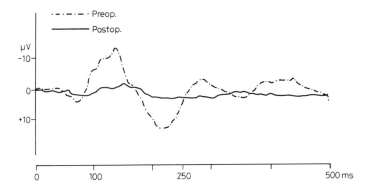

Fig. 1. Pre- and postoperative recording of REP in the same animal (angular acceleration 7.5 °/s², clockwise rotation).

were substantially reduced: P2–P3, 4.5 µV (SD 2.9 µV); P3–P4, 5.0 µV (SD 3.5 µV). Mechanical and myogenic artifacts could be excluded by firm fixation of the animals inside the rotating drum.

Discussion

Postoperative potentials appear to be strikingly reduced in amplitude if compared with the normal. This reduction becomes particularly obvious in the 'late' peaks P3 and P4 which are significantly flattened in the arithmetic average and could not even be identified in many single recordings. In addition to low amplitude, the latencies of P3 and P4 show a much more pronounced scattering in labyrinthectomized rabbits which indicates that they might well be coincidental. With the two 'late' latencies (between 150 and 250 ms) being severely affected by labyrinthectomy, it seems likely that they represent a cortical potential caused by the afferent vestibular fibers.

We postulate further that the 'early' peaks P1 and P2 (between 50 and 100 ms) which show a more constant occurrence, even after labyrinthectomy, can be attributed to afferent sources other than the vestibular system, such as epicritic or proprioceptive receptors in the body's periphery, commonly called 'somatosensory'. We believe that those early potentials which are less affected by destruction of the labyrinth might give a clue to the phenomenon of almost entire habituation following total loss of the labyrinthine sense of balance, which we witnessed in our rabbits several weeks after surgery.

Although the regaining of balance after bilateral transection of the eighth cranial nerve was first observed as early as 1883 by Bechterew [1883] in dogs and has been a fortunate experience for many an ENT surgeon, a plausible explanation for this fascinating fact has not yet been found. Using an animal model such as the rabbit, our microsurgical approach to the inner ear is extremely useful in producing chronic loss of labyrinthine function and can help clarify this situation. We found that because of the similarity with the human REP, the rabbit lends itself ideally to further research into vestibular and other related potentials.

References

Bechterew, W.: Ergebnisse der Durchschneidung des Nervus acusticus, nebst Erörterung der Bedeutung der semicirculären Canäle für das Körpergleichgewicht. Pflügers Arch. ges. Physiol. *30* (1883).

Hofferberth, B.: Evoked potentials to rotatory stimulation. Acta oto-lar., suppl. 406, pp. 134–136 (1984).

Kornhuber, H.; Da Fonseca, J.: Optovestibular integration in the cat's cortex: a study of sensory convergence on cortical neurons; in Bender, The oculomotor system, pp. 239–279 (Hoeber, New York 1964).

Ödkvist, L.; Rubin, A.; Schwarz, D.; Fredrickson, J.: Vestibular cortical projection in the rabbit. J. comp. Neurol. *149:* 117–120 (1973).

B. Hofferberth, MD, Department of Neurology, University of Münster, D-4400 Münster (FRG)

Adv. Oto-Rhino-Laryng., vol. 41, pp. 210–215 (Karger, Basel 1988)

Head Rotation Evoked EEG Responses Are Governed by Rate of Angular Acceleration Change

H.C. Hansen, W.H. Zangemeister, K. Kunze

Neurological University Clinic Hamburg, Hamburg, FRG

Introduction and Methods

Cortical evoked potentials (EP) are well known for monitoring of various sensory pathways, for the vestibular system so far no standard testing has been established although cortical vestibular projections in parietal regions and the motor-somatosensory border zone could be demonstrated in mammals [Oedkvist et al., 1977]. Both regions have been shown to receive extensive proprioceptor input which converges at different levels (vestibular nuclei, thalamus, cerebral cortex) with the afferent vestibular (vest.) signal [Deecke et al., 1977; Fredrickson et al., 1966; Oedkvist et al., 1975]. Therefore, an experimental paradigm of active head rotation providing both input modalities was designed, contrasting with previous studies, where mostly passive whole body rotations had served as stimuli with lower peak acceleration values.

The data presented here were obtained from 10 normal subjects who had performed 400 alternating fast head rotations while five EEG, EOG and head accelerations (ACC) were recorded. Care was taken for movement artifacts (needle electrodes, preamplification of EEG on the subject's head) and counter-rotational eye movements were suppressed by an earlier described technique [Hansen et al., 1986]. After visual inspection of single trials, four samples of 36 movements, representing the fastest and slowest in both directions, were selected out of the 400 recorded head movements and used in a regular averaging programme triggering on the ascending part of the head acceleration trace.

Results

The EP on a basis of 36 single trials showed a typical four-peak pattern as described earlier [Zangemeister et al., 1986] (fig. 1). Out of the four peaks, the

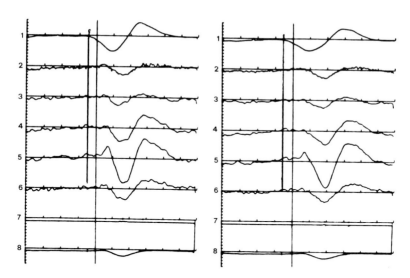

Fig. 1. Typical head rotation evoked responses for 36 rotations to the left in the same subject. Each record shows acceleration on trace 1, EOG on trace 8 and EP on traces 2–6, in the order Fz, Cz, Pz, P4, P3. Calibrations are 10,000 °/s² for 1. 25 μV for 2–6 and 5° for trace 8, upward deflection indicating leftward movement or negativity, respectively. Responses to slower rotations (lower peak ACC, on the right) show lower amplitudes, maximum response at parietal recording sites.

most consistent were N2 at 178 ms and P1 at 295 ms, obtained for rotations in both directions and appeared without side asymmetries over both parietal recording sites. The lowest amplitudes (AMP) found were usually frontal, while maximum EP were detected over centroparietal regions. As well as latency (LAT), amplitude did not alter significantly with change of rotational direction, which is consistent with anatomical reports of bilateral ascending vestibular-kinesthetic pathways.

Comparison of slower and faster rotation EP showed that all subjects with one exception reacted in a uniform way to increasing head acceleration, namely acceleration increase being associated with higher peak-to-peak amplitude and shorter latencies (p <0.01 and 0.005). The change in latency to acceleration change was constant in all subjects (linear regression correlation coefficient r=0.85) though absolute latency was not correlated with absolute accelerations (fig. 2). Similarly, for the N2–P1 peak-to-peak amplitude an intraindividual increase was found when EP of faster movements were compared with those of slower ones. Normalized amplitude change (i.e.

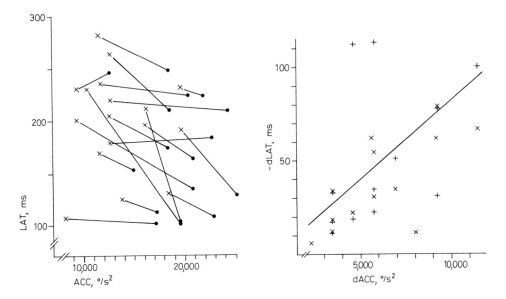

Fig. 2. On the right, pairs of EP representing fast and slow movement responses of the same subject are shown in terms of N2 and P1 latency and corresponding acceleration, showing a decrease of latency with a rise in acceleration. The left part shows that a change of latency (dLAT) increases proportionally with a change of acceleration (dACC) for both N2 (×) and P1 (+) peak latencies.

change in amplitude divided by the lower amplitude observed) was proportional to normalized acceleration change in a log-log plot, with $r = 0.78$ (fig. 3).

It must be stressed, however, that the interindividual comparison yielded no correlation between absolute latency and amplitude values on one side and head accelerations on the other side, although a tendency for relative high amplitude and low latency in faster movements was noticed. Therefore, shifting of latency and amplitude must be viewed on a purely individual basis, reflecting central pathway reactions to the multimodal stimulation used in this experimental paradigm.

This study showed that the known EP to head rotation depends on the peak acceleration of the head used, pointing to the semicircular canals as an acceleration-detecting organ. The maximum activity being located over centro-parietal regions suggests further topographically oriented studies to concentrate there.

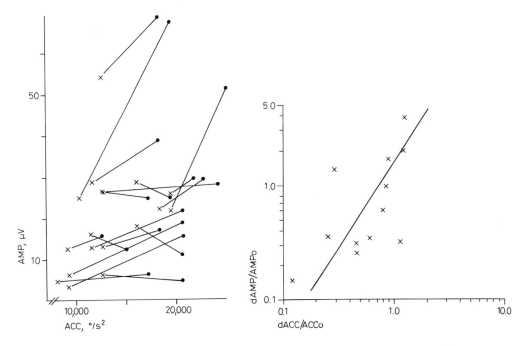

Fig. 3. Compared to figure 2, the relation between amplitude and acceleration is shown. On the right, the rise in amplitude (N2–P1) is demonstrated for most of the subjects investigated, and on the left a linear increase is shown for normalized change in amplitude (dAMP/AMPo) for all subjects.

Discussion

Control experiments done before with active trunk and wrist rotations [Hansen et al., 1986] that yielded only low late activation rule out a pure proprioceptive equivalent of the potential found. Further evidence comes from experiments using voluntary finger movements [Shibasaki et al., 1980] where a reduction in amplitude was noticed when passive to active movements were compared.

Considering a dominant role for the vestibular input, the underlying process starting with N1 at 66 and N2 at 178 ms, does not reflect the discharge of primary vestibular projections, for lower conduction times would be expected. We therefore suggest that areas of secondary or higher order, as might be related to posture sensation or control, are involved as the underlying generators. There, the mechanism producing latency and amplitude shifting could be a threshold sensitivity at any level of the ascending pathway that reacts only after a certain acceleration is reached, in that way discharging earlier in faster rotational movements. Alternatively, a sensitivity to the derivative of acceleration that has a higher and earlier reached peak in faster movements could also explain these results. Taken together with our results concerning proprioceptive stimulation, it seems that synchronous proprioception facilitates and produces the relatively high peaks compared to other studies.

The patterns found in other (passive) rotational paradigms also seem to show a correlation between the response and the underlying acceleration stimulus [Hood et al., 1985; Hofferberth, 1984] with an enlargement of the response in length (i.e. latency) and a decrease in amplitude in slower rotational dynamic conditions. Moreover, Boehmer et al. [1983] reported that passive head rotation EP had shown about twice the amplitude of a whole body rotation response in their rhesus monkey study.

In earlier studies, we reported that EP of patients with vestibular deficits had shown side asymmetries or general amplitude reductions. We expect, especially in the latter group, that testing for EP shifting might yield important information for clinical diagnosis.

References

Boehmer, A.; Henn, V.; Lehmann, D.: Vestibular evoked potentials in the awake rhesus monkey. Adv. Oto-Rhino-Laryng., vol. 30, pp. 54–57 (Karger, Basel 1983).

Deecke, L.; Schwarz, D.W.F.; Fredrickson, J.M.: Vestibular responses in the rhesus monkey ventroposterior thalamus. II. Vestibulo-proprioceptive converence at thalamic neurons. Exp. Brain Res. *30:* 219–232 (1977).

Fredrickson, J.M.; Schwarz, D.W.F.; Kornhuber, H.H.: Convergence and interaction of vestibular and deep somatic afferents upon neurons in the vestibular nuclei in the cat. Acta oto-lar. *61:* 168–188 (1966).

Hansen, H.C.; Zangemeister, W.H.; Kunze, K.: Cortical activity in response to voluntary stimulation of vestibular, cervical and brachial proprioceptors; in Kunze, Zangemeister, Arlt, Clinical problems of brainstem disorders, pp. 213–217 (Thieme, Stuttgart 1986).

Hofferberth. B.: Evoked potentials to rotary stimulation. Acta oto-lar., suppl. 406, pp. 134–136 (1984).

Hood, J.D.; Kayan, A.: Observations upon the evoked responses to natural vestibular stimulation. Electroenceph. clin. Neurophysiol. *62:* 266–276 (1985).

Oedkvist, L.M.; Larsby, B.; Fredrickson, J.M.: Projection of the vestibular nerve to the SI arm field in the cerebral cortex of the cat. Acta oto-lar. *79:* 88–95 (1975).

Oedkvist, L.M.; Liedgren, S.R.C.; Aschan, G.: Cerebral cortex and vestibular nerve. Adv. Oto-Rhino-Laryng., vol. 22, pp. 125–135 (Karger, Basel 1977).

Shibasaki, H.; Barrett, G.; Halliday, E.; Halliday, A.M.: Cortical potentials following voluntary and passive finger movements. Electroenceph. clin. Neurophysiol. *50:* 201–213 (1980).

Zangemeister, W.H.; Phlebs, U.; Huefner, G.; Kunze, K.: Active head turning correlated cerebral potentials. Acta oto-lar. *101:* 403–415 (1986).

H.C. Hansen, Neurological University Clinic, Martinistrasse 52, D-2000 Hamburg (FRG)

Adv. Oto-Rhino-Laryng., vol. 41, pp. 216–223 (Karger, Basel 1988)

Magnetic Resonance Imaging in the Diagnosis of Lesions of the Central Vestibular Structures

A. Pirodda[a], *G. Brayda*[b], *C. Trevisan*[b], *E. Pirodda*[a]

[a]Clinica Otorinolaringologica dell'Università di Bologna;
[b]Centro Diagnostico Città di Bologna, Italy

Magnetic resonance imaging (MRI) seems to have already found a privileged place, among the modern procedures involving computerized imaging, in the clinical study of the CNS, in particular of the structures of the posterior fossa [3, 5, 7]. The influence of bony structures on the quality of images is practically negligible, the procedure does not require the use of contrast media and, not least, does not expose the subject to ionizing radiations. Furthermore, the resolution power of MRI is substantially higher than that of comparable procedures, thus allowing for the possibility of obtaining more detailed information. On the other hand, clinical experience, which up to the present time is relatively limited, points out some difficulties in the interpretation of results. Mechanisms essentially different from those involved in traditional procedures are at the basis of the production of MR images, and matching them with clinical symptomatology may at times prove to be a difficult task [1].

In the present situation, another essential fact must be kept in mind, i.e. that the present procedures of MRI are based upon the signals produced by the H nuclei. Images obtained by this technique, therefore, necessarily tend to emphasize aspects concerning structures or processes (fluids, edema), the presence of which implies a high relative content of H protons [1]. Also it must be mentioned that the procedure lends itself to promising developments and integrations, as extensively illustrated in recent reviews [2, 6].

In conclusion, a number of reasons justify a particular interest in the subject on the part of the clinician. As far as we were able to find out, morphological aspects in MRI of structures pertaining to the central vestibular pathways have not been a subject for systematic investigation in normal individuals.

Material and Methods

Ten normal healthy young persons served as subjects for a morphological orientative study. Due to the limited availability of the MRI equipment, only a limited number of pathological cases could be examined. Cases were selected on the basis of the clinical characteristics of the vestibular symptomatology. Preference was given to patients whose symptomatology was exclusively or predominantly, at least in the initial stage, of vestibular nature, and of presumptive central origin. Ordinary vestibular tests and the rest of the clinico-neurological picture did not provide sufficiently complete information for a reliable diagnosis of these patients. Obviously, MRI examination could be expected to provide essential data in some cases, whilst in others it would have in any case represented an extremely interesting objective contribution to the diagnosis, to be evaluated in correlation with the characteristics of the vestibular symptomatology.

As for the technical details, a superconducting Philips MRI system was used. In the investigation of normal subjects images were T1-weighted and generated with a spin echo pulse sequence using an echo time (TE) of 30 ms and a repetition time (TR) of 350 ms. The examination was performed on pathological subjects with a spin echo pulse sequence using a TE of 50 ms and a TR of 1,500 ms and with a multi-echo sequence, in order to obtain a predominantly T1-weighted first echo and predominantly T2-weighted second echo.

Results

The study of 10 normal subjects, through examination of planes corresponding to the vestibular nuclear complex and brain stem vestibular pathways, provided images which show these structures in as yet unmatched details (fig. 1, 2) as well as in their individual variations. Some of our observations on pathological cases deserve to be briefly illustrated.

A characteristic example concerning the first group of patients (a neurological picture where vestibular symptomatology was predominant, or at least one of the initial manifestations) is illustrated in figures 3 and 4.

The female patient, aged 22, had been suddenly struck by an acute neurological symptomatology consisting of vertigo, paresis of the VIIth nerve and right hemiparesis. Within 48 h the symptoms were partially regressed. After one month any sign of neurological involvement completely disappeared. The patient is still symptom-free up to the present time. MRI corresponding to one month (fig. 3) and 2 months (fig. 4) following the onset of the clinical symptomatology show a voluminous lesion in the bulbo-pontine anterior region and document a tendency to regression which parallels the regression of the clinical symptoms. The nature of this process remains unknown, in the absence of any other source of information (CT was thought to provide no additional information).

Two cases deserve to be mentioned in the second group of patients where the vestibular symptomatology was, at least for some time, the only clinical manifestation of

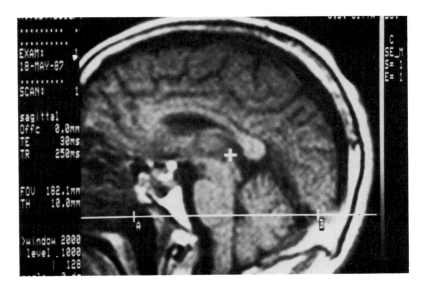

Fig. 1. Normal subject, lateral projection. Line shows the level of axial projection.

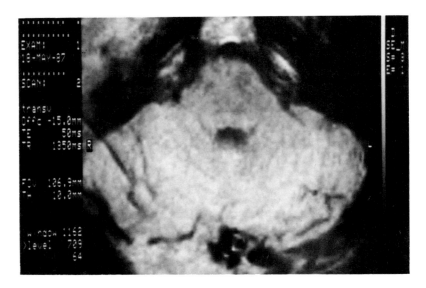

Fig. 2. Normal subject, axial projection.

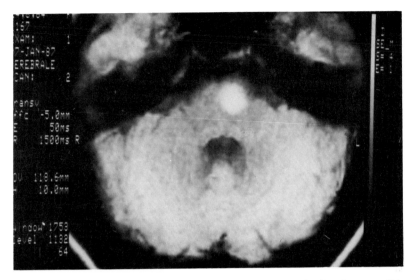

Fig. 3. A 22-year-old female patient. MRI performed one month after the onset of the symptomatology, axial projection.

neurological disorder. They may be considered a significant demonstration of the extremely important role that NMR may play in the diagnosis of lesions of the CNS involving the vestibular structures. The first observation concerns a female patient, aged 34, whose symptomatology (dating back about 2 years) consisted of vertigo, nausea, vomiting and headache. Brain stem auditory evoked potentials showed only a reduced voltage of the main deflections, visual evoked potentials similarly showed reduced voltages and slightly increased latencies. Vestibular examination revealed a spontaneous right beating nystagmus, some minor qualitative abnormalities, occasionally dissociation phenomena, both qualitative and quantitative, in the ny reflex responses following rotoacceleratory as well as caloric stimulations. In character the vestibular function, however, was essentially preserved.

Fixation optokinetic nystagmus was markedly reduced — CT scanning gave negative results 4 months before our examination. MRI demonstrated the presence of some limited focal lesions in the paramedian subcortical areas of both parietal lobes and in the right semi-oval center (fig. 5, 6).

A second typical observation is provided by another 42-year-old female whose symptomatology consisted only of vertigo and nausea, showing a tendency to a progressive worsening. Vestibular tests gave evidence of a condition of imbalance, with a tendency to falling to the right and ataxic gait. MRI showed a relatively limited lesion involving the vestibular nuclear area, to the right of the IVth ventricle, in the region of the lateral recess (fig. 7). In the following months the diagnosis of multiple sclerosis was established.

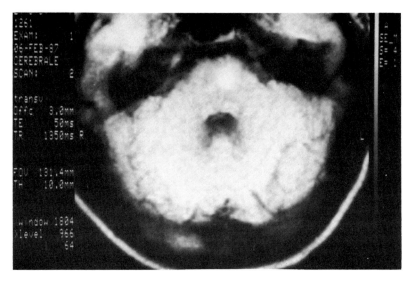

Fig. 4. The same patient, MRI performed 2 months after the onset of the symptomatology.

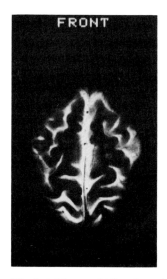

Fig. 5. A 34-year-old female patient, axi . projection.

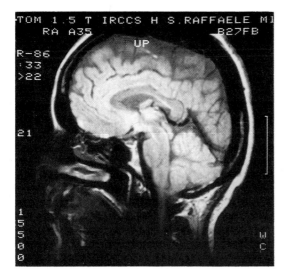

Fig. 6. The same patient, sagittal projection.

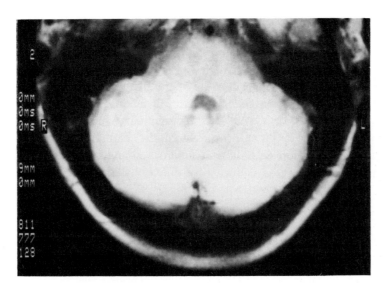

Fig. 7. A 42-year-old female patient, axial projection.

Comment

MRI procedures have been applied for clinical purposes only in relatively recent times. Much has still to be learnt about the data it is capable of providing, through the variety of its technologies, and about the morphology and biochemistry of CNS structures in normal as well as in different pathological situations.

It is sufficiently clear, however, that MRI, even at its present stage of development, in spite of its present limitations, is destined to play a fundamental role in the clinical investigation of the structures of the CNS. Foreseeable developments promise a better insight also into the metabolic processes occurring within different regions of the CNS in vivo. Studies on individual variations within normal ranges may lead to findings of some clinical significance.

As for lesions of the vestibular pathways, at present, on the basis of our own observations as illustrated by our selected cases, the following conclusions may be drawn:

(1) In addition to its complementary role in the best definition of a number of lesions of the CNS, MRI shows decisive importance in the diagnosis of some cases where any other clinical investigation proved inconclusive. Early detection of foci of multiple sclerosis [4, 8, 9], as well as of other more or less limited focal lesions of a lesser known nature, seems to be greatly improved by this procedure, as indicated also by the aforementioned examples.

(2) MRI appears to provide/promise, through its hitherto unsurpassed capability of providing original detailed and dynamic morphological data, an extremely valuable contribution to solving difficulties and uncertainties in the diagnosis of a consistent number of clinical conditions where a vestibular component is involved. Vestibular symptomatology, occurring either isolated or in the context of a more or less complex neurological symptomatology, can be much more satisfactorily understood and correlated with data provided by the clinical tests during the different stages of evolution of the lesion.

References

1   Biller, J.; Adams, H.P., Jr.; Dunn, V.; Simmons, Z.; Jacoby, C.G.: Dichotomy between clinical findings and MR abnormalities in pontine infarction. J. Comput. assist. Tomogr. *10:* 379–385 (1986).

2   Gadian, D.G.: Nuclear magnetic resonance and its applications to living systems. (Clarendon Press, Oxford 1982).

3   Han, J.S.; Bonstelle, C.T.; Kaufman, B.; Benson, J.E.; Alfidi, R.J.; Clampitt, M.; Van Dyke, C.; Huss, R.G.: Magnetic resonance imaging in the evaluation of the brainstem. Radiology *150:* 705–712 (1984).

4   Jacobs, L.; Kinkel, W.R.; Polachini, I.; Kinkel, R.P.: Correlations of nuclear magnetic resonance imaging, computerized tomography, and clinical profile in multiple sclerosis. Neurology *36:* 27–34 (1986).

5   Kirshner, H.S.; Tsai, S.I.; Runge, V.M.; et al.: Magnetic resonance imaging and other techniques in the diagnosis of multiple sclerosis. Archs Neurol. *42:* 859–863 (1985).

6   Lauterbur, P.C.; Dias, D.H.M.; Rudin, A.M.: Augmentation of tissue water proton relaxation rates in vivo by addition of paramagnetic ions; in Dutton, Leigh, Scarpa, Frontiers of biological energetics, pp. 752–759 (Academic Press, New York 1980).

7   Leboldus, G.M.; Savoury, L.W.; Carr, T.J.; Nicholson, R.L.: Magnetic resonance imaging: a review of basic principles and potential use in otolaryngology. J. Otolaryngol. *15:* 273–278 (1986).

8   Pirodda, A.; Rinaldi Ceroni, A.; Ambrosetto, P.: Contributo della RM alla topodiagnosi di sindromi vertiginose di origine centrale. Acta oto-rhinol. ital. *6:* 423–430 (1986).

9   Rumbach, L.; Caires, M.,C.; Warter, J.M.; Collard, M.; Sheiber, C.; Gounot, D.; Dumitresco, B.; Chambron, J.: Contribution à l'étude de l'imagerie par résonance magnétique nucléaire du proton dans la sclérose en plaques. Apport d'une séquence spin-echo multiple. Revue neurol. *141:* 583–586 (1985).

A. Pirodda, MD, Clinica Otorinolaringologica dell'Università di Bologna, Via Massarenti 9, I-40138 Bologna (Italy)

Adv. Oto-Rhino-Laryng., vol. 41, pp. 224–228 (Karger, Basel 1988)

Posterior Fossa: Correlations between Anatomical Slices and Magnetic Resonance Imaging

E. Vitte[a,c], *M. Baulac*[a], *D. Dormont*[b], *D. Hasboun*[a],
J.J. Sarcy[d], *G. Freyss*[c]

[a]Laboratoire d'Anatomie, CHU Pitié-Salpêtrière; [b]Service de Neuroradiologie,
CHU Pitié-Salpêtrière; [c]Chaire de Clinique ORL, Hôpital Lariboisière;
[d]Laboratoire d'Anatomie, CHU Necker, Paris, France

Small structures, especially cochleovestibular or oculomotor nuclei, are difficult to localize on magnetic resonance imaging (MRI). Their topography is more accurately identified on serial brain slices. A good correlation between brain imaging and anatomical studies could help in diagnosis of small CNS lesions.

Materials and Methods

Anatomical Slices. Serial slices from skull and brain, 3 mm thick, have been performed according to the method of Delmas and Pertuiset [2]. Planes of sections have been determined with bony structures; the axial plane was the horizontal plane defined by the line passing between the superior edge of the external auditory canal and the lowest point of the inferior orbital ridge. The frontal and sagittal planes were perpendicular to the axial one.

MR Images. MR images were obtained on a super-conducting MR imager (CGR Magniscan 5000) operating at a field strength of 0.5 T. Scans were obtained using the inversion-recovery pulse sequence with an inversion time (TI) of 450 ms, repetition time (TR) of 1,500 ms and echo time (TE) of 28 ms. In each plane, identical to the anatomical one, a set of a-mm-thick slices was obtained first; then a second set was obtained after a a/2-mm translation, in order to get a slice every a/2-mm. Image reconstruction was performed on healthy volunteers by 2D Fourier transformation onto a 256 × 256 matrix.

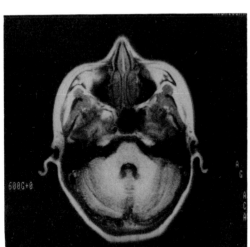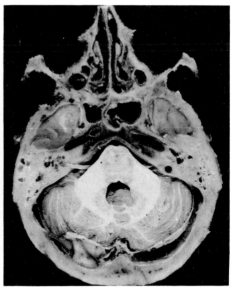

a

b

Fig. 1. Axial plane. *a* MRI; *b* brain slice. Acousticofacial nerves are well seen.

Results

Axial Plane

The axial planes (horizontal and OM planes) are the most useful to study posterior fossa.

Vestibulocerebellum and Vestibular Nuclei. The nodulus is protruding in the fourth ventricle cavity on the slices passing through the upper medulla. Flocculus is the most lateral component of the cerebellopontine angle (fig. 1).

The nuclear complex comprises the four well-known nuclei: superior, lateral, medial and inferior. They are localized at the lateral edge of the floor of the fourth ventricle (at the pons-medulla oblongata junction). We can only presume their localization on our MR images.

Cerebellopontine Angle and Internal Auditory Canal. The acousticofacial nerves are seen in the internal auditory canal and in the cerebellopontine angle as well. They emerge from the brain stem between the medulla and the pons in front of the flocculus. On MRI the signal is homogeneous.

Oculomotor Nuclei. The sixth nucleus is easy to localize on the slices through the pons due to its projection on the floor of the fourth ventricle near the midline (eminentia teres). The landmarks to delineate the third nerve nuclei are the periaqueductal gray matter and the superior colliculi. Both are seen on MRI. The medial longitudinal fasciculus (MLF) is a dorsally situated bundle of fibres arising from abducens nuclei (sixth nerve) and projecting on oculomotor nuclei (third nerve) on the opposite side. The MLF carries various ascending fibres from the vestibular nuclei and descending fibres from the pontine reticular formation. On axial planes and on brain slices it can be localized near the midline.

Frontal Plane

Vestibulocerebellum. On brain slices, the acousticofacial nerves are clearly seen when crossing the flocculus. Nodulus can be visualized on posterior slices with internal cerebellar nuclei.

Cerebellopontine Angle and Internal Auditory Canal. On MRI, the frontal plane is a good way to see small acoustic neuromas, but for the neurovascular bundle the coronal section is not as reliable [5].

Oculomotor Nuclei. On the same slice, we can see the four colliculi; the periaqueductal gray is longitudinally cut (fig. 2). This plane appears to be useful to study the fourth ventricle and vestibulocerebellum.

Sagittal Plane

As the flocculus is seen on the lateral slices, the nodulus is well delineated on sagittal sections since it constitutes a part of the roof of the fourth ventricle. This plane shows the three pairs of cerebellar peduncles.

Oculomotor Nuclei (fig. 3). Since the oculomotor nuclei can be localized near the midline, the MLF is sometimes visible when it appears as 'a pseudo-MLF hyperintensity'. It is a strictly midline, linear area of hyperintensity just anterior to the aqueduct and fourth ventricle [1].

Conclusion

The MR sequences that are widely used for the demonstration of brain lesions (T2 weighted) are often of lower anatomical definition than those

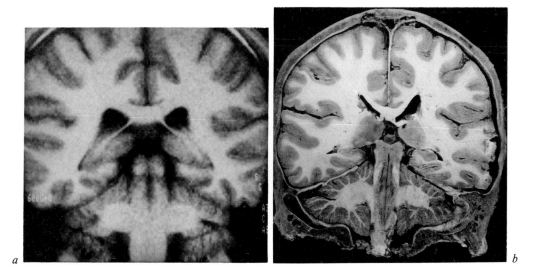

Fig. 2. Coronal plane. *a* MRI; *b* brain slice. Periaqueductal gray matter is cut longitudinally.

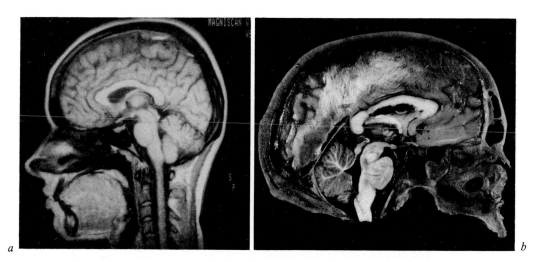

Fig. 3. Sagittal plane. *a* MRI; *b* brain slice. MLF is seen on brain slice.

used for the present study. It then appears very important to possess a large base of serial cross-sectional data concerning posterior fossa which can be used as anatomical references.

References

1   Atlas, W.S.; et al.: Internuclear ophthalmoplegia — MR anatomic correlation. AJNR 8: 243 (1987).
2   Delmas, A.; Pertuiset, B.: Craniocerebral topometry in man. (Masson, Paris 1959).
3   Carpenter, M.B.: Human neuroanatomy; 7th ed. (Williams & Wilkins, Baltimore 1976).
4   Nieuwenhuys, R.; Voogd, J.; Van Huijzen, C.H.: The human central nervous system: a synopsis and atlas; 2nd ed. (Springer, Berlin 1981).
5   Vignaud, J.; Jardin, C.; Rosen, L.: The ear. Diagnostic imaging. (Masson, New York 1986).

E. Vitte, MD, Laboratoire d'Anatomie, CHU Pitié-Salpêtrière, 105 Bd de l'Hôpital, F-75013 Paris (France)

Adv. Oto-Rhino-Laryng., vol. 41, pp. 229–230 (Karger, Basel 1988)

Vascular Disease as a Cause of Vertigo and Hearing Loss: The Role of 'Normal' Alcohol Consumption

H.H. Kornhuber

Department of Neurology, Ulm University, Ulm , FRG

Many cases of tinnitus, sudden hearing loss and vestibular 'neuronitis' are of vascular origin [8]. The cardiovascular risk factors play a major role in labyrinthine as in cerebral vascular disease, although arteritis as a cause of cerebrovascular (and possibly of labyrinthine) disease occurs more frequently than hitherto assumed [4]. When an inflammatory disease is excluded, the acute case of hearing or vestibular loss should be treated in a similar way as a stroke with a lipophilic calcium antagonist (flunarizine), aspirin and hemodilution if necessary. However, for both treatment and prevention, the cardiovascular risk factors should be reduced. In this respect it is not recognized enough that, besides nicotine, the single major cause of obesity [5], hyperlipidemia [1], type II diabetes [6] and high blood pressure [7] is the 'normal' (daily moderate) alcohol consumption in the human male today. Alcohol damages the insulin receptors [5] and thus causes hyperinsulinemia [6] which in turn blocks the lipolysis (leading to obesity even without increased caloric intake) and enhances the renal sodium reabsorption [2] which causes high blood pressure. Furthermore, hyperinsulinemia is a major cause of atherosclerosis [9]. Even in apparently healthy young males with 'normal' daily alcohol consumption, hepatic steatosis with hyperinsulinemia is a very common finding today [3]; this is positively correlated with overweight, hypertriglyceridemia, hypercholesterinemia and high blood pressure. Moreover 'normal' alcohol consumption [5] is the most common cause of type II diabetes in the human male [1, 6]. To reduce overweight and to normalize serum lipids, glucose metabolism and blood pressure, it is not enough to prescribe drugs: to help the patient more carefully it is indispensable to cure him of the habit of daily alcohol consumption. Regarding cerebrovascular disease this treatment is more helpful than any other [1], and because of the similarity of the cerebral and the labyrinthine blood supply regulations this is probably valid for the inner ear.

References

1   Altmann, J.; Kornhuber, A.W.; Kornhuber, H.H.: Stroke: cardiovascular risk factors and the quantitative effects of dietary treatment on them. Eur. Neurol. *26:* 90–99 (1987).
2   DeFronzo, R.A.: Insulin and renal sodium handling: clinical implications. Int. J. Obes. *5.* suppl. 1, pp. 93–104 (1981).
3   Henkler, C.; Kornhuber, A.; Kornhuber, H.H.; Scheben, B.; Molz, K.H.; Maier, V.; Swobodnik, W.; Wechsler, J.G.: Am Anfang des Weges zum Schlaganfall: Insulinrezeptor-Schädigung durch Alkohol und Fettleber-Hyperinsulinismus bei jungen Männern. Dt. med. Wschr. *112:* 157–158 (1987).
4   Hülser, P.J.; Kornhuber, H.H.; Risotto, R.: Schlaganfall und Herzinfarkt durch Arteriitis. Dt. med. Wschr. *110:* 1753–1754 (1985).
5   Kornhuber, H.H.: 'Normaler' Alkoholkonsum — eine der Ursachen von Bluthochdruck, Adipositas und Atherosklerose. 'Normal' alcohol consumption, a cause of high blood pressure, obesity and atherosclerosis. Schweiz. Rdsch. Med. Praxis *75:* 1577–1579 (1986).
6   Kornhuber, H.H.; Lisson, G.; Suschka-Sauermann, L.: Adipositas und Artherosklerose als spezifisch-toxische Alkoholfolgen. Öff. Gesundh.-Wes. *47:* 488–496 (1985).
7   Kornhuber, H.H.; Lisson, G.; Suschka-Sauermann, L.: Alcohol and obesity: a new look at high blood pressure and stroke. An epidemiological study in preventive neurology. Eur. Arch. Psychiat. Neurol. Sci. *234:* 357–362 (1985).
8   Kornhuber, H.H.; Waldecker, G.: Akute isolierte periphere Vestibularisstörungen. Arch. Ohr.-Nas.-KehlkHeilk. *173:* 340 (1958).
9   Stout, R.-W.: Diabetes and atherosclerosis — the role of insulin. Diabetologia *16:* 141–150 (1979).

H.H. Kornhuber, MD, Department of Neurology, Ulm University,
D-7900 Ulm (FRG)

Adv. Oto-Rhino-Laryng., vol. 41, pp. 231–234 (Karger, Basel 1988)

Noninvasive Ultrasound Investigation of Cerebral Vessels in the Case of Vertigo and Dizziness

B. Widder, H.H. Kornhuber, A. Kornhuber

University of Ulm, Ulm, FRG

Stenoses and occlusions of the brain supplying arteries are not uncommon causes for vertigo and dizziness. In a few cases, these symptoms can even be the only precursor preceding a stroke. Therefore, such occlusive disease must be taken into consideration when attempting to treat patients with vestibular, cochlear and vertebrobasilar symptoms, especially if there is no sign of inflammatory labyrinthine disorder.

Today this can be done by investigating the cerebral vessels by means of noninvasive ultrasound technique. *Extracranial Doppler sonography* enables one to estimate the blood flow velocity in the carotid and vertebral artery by use of a small hand-held probe, which can be moved along the vessels. This method is suitable for the reliable detection of higher grade stenoses and occlusions [1]. Hand-held Doppler sonography, however, fails in hemodynamically noncritical, lower grade stenoses. Such stenoses can be readily investigated by *B-mode imaging* [2]. On the other hand, the B-scan frequently fails in severe occlusive diseases because of imaging problems. Therefore, *duplex sonography* as a combination of both methods is the best choice, giving information about the morphological as well as the hemodynamical situation (fig. 1) [3, 6].

As in the carotid artery, Doppler sonography is also able to estimate flow disturbances in the vertebral artery. This may be of special interest in the case of subclavian steal effects with retrograde flow in the vertebral artery due to a high grade stenosis or an occlusion of the proximal subclavian artery. By use of *transnuchal Doppler sonography* through the foramen magnum also the basilar artery can be followed in its course. This enables one to detect basilar artery stenoses and occlusions.

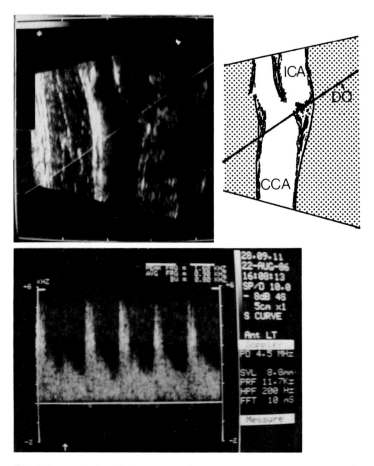

Fig. 1. Internal carotid artery stenosis with a diameter reduction of about 70% as shown by duplex sonography. Above: The B-mode image of the carotid bifurcation demonstrating a stenosis at the origin of the internal carotid artery. Below: The pulsatile blood flow velocity measured by Doppler technique at the maximum of the stenosis.

Finally, recently available *transcranial Doppler sonography* extends the diagnostic possibilities on other intracranial vessels [5]. By transtemporal insonation of the great basal arteries it is possible to detect Doppler flow signals from the middle cerebral artery, the distal portion of the internal carotid artery, the anterior cerebral artery and the proximal portion of the posterior cerebral artery. By combination with short-term digital compression of the common carotid artery the patency of the circle of Willis can be assessed and intracranial steal effects can be verified (fig. 2).

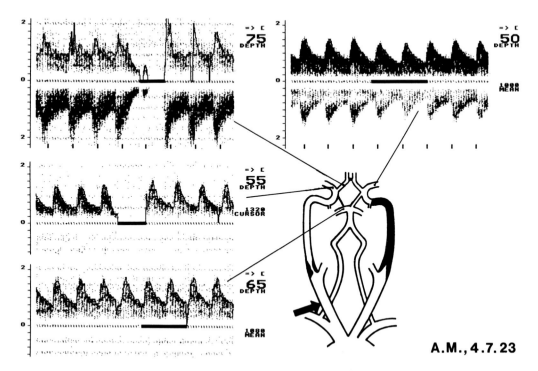

Fig. 2. Right carotid artery stenosis and contralateral occlusion in a patient suffering from frequent attacks of vertigo as the only clinical symptom. Compression of the right common carotid artery (—) results in an unmeasurable flow velocity in the ipsilateral middle and anterior cerebral artery. The flow in the left middle cerebral artery and the posterior cerebral artery is not affected, demonstrating hypoplasia of both the anterior and the right posterior communicating artery. Therefore, a surgical removal of the stenosis did not seem to be helpful.

In addition, the sufficiency of intracranial collateralization can also be quantified. In the case of an intact circle of Willis, even a total occlusion of the internal carotid artery may have no hemodynamic effect on the cerebral circulation. However, in the case of hypoplasia of the intracranial collaterals, a sufficient cerebral blood flow can only be maintained by dilation of the intracerebral arterioles. This results in a loss of cerebral autoregulation, and sudden drops in blood pressure may cause ischemic events. The capacity of the cerebral arterioles to dilate further can be tested by using CO_2 inhalation during Doppler registration (Doppler CO_2 test) [4].

In summary, recently available ultrasound methods like duplex scanning and transcranial Doppler sonography are able to detect stenoses and occlusions of the great brain supplying extra- and intracranial arteries in patients with vertigo and dizziness. The investigations are completely noninvasive, and hemodynamic tests help to decide whether surgical treatment of an occlusive disease may be efficient. The method, so far mainly used by neurologists, is also suitable for use by otologists.

References

1   Widder, B.; Kornhuber, H.H.: Zuverlässigkeit und Grenzen dopplersonographischer Untersuchungen der kranialen Arterien. Fortschr. Röntgenstr. *135:* 80–84 (1981).

2   Widder, B.; Kornhuber, H.H.: Möglichkeiten und Grenzen der hochauflösenden B-Bild-Sonographie an der A. carotis. Fortschr. Röntgenstr. *141:* 683–689 (1984).

3   Widder, B.: Ultraschalluntersuchungen der hirnversorgenden Arterien — Bedeutung für Diagnostik und Therapie. Hämostaseologie *6:* 216–224 (1986).

4   Widder, B.; Paulat, K.; Hackspacher, J.; Mayr, E.: Transcranial Doppler CO_2-test for the detection of hemodynamically critical carotid artery stenoses and occlusions. Eur. Arch. Psychiat. Neurol. Sci. *236:* 162–168 (1986).

5   Widder, B. (ed.): Transkranielle Dopplersonographie bei zerebrovaskulären Erkrankungen. Stellenwert für Diagnostik in Therapie (Springer, Heidelberg 1987).

6   Widder, B.; Paulat, K.; Kreutzer, C.; Ott, F.: Is Duplex scanning able to estimate the embolic risk of ICA stenoses? J. cardiovasc. Ultrasonogr. *5:* 13 (1986).

B. Widder, MD, PhD, University of Ulm, D-7900 Ulm (FRG)

Adv. Oto-Rhino-Laryng., vol. 41, pp. 235–238 (Karger, Basel 1988)

Quantified EEG Cartography, Computerized Electro-Oculography in Hemodynamic Vertebrobasilar Insufficiency, Modifications Induced by Vertebral Artery Compression

C. Sebban[a], *E. Vitte*[b], *G. Rancurel*[c],
K. Le Roch[a], *G. Benkemoun*[a], *N. Tzourio*[c], *G. Freyss*[b]

[a]Hôpital Charles Foix, Ivry; [b]Chaire de Clinique ORL, Hôpital Lariboisière;
[c]Service de Neurologie, CHU Pitié-Salpêtrière, Paris, France

Diagnosis of hemodynamic vertebrobasilar insufficiency (VBIPH) remains difficult and clinical [1, 2]. The authors sought a noninvasive method to prove the diagnosis and developed vertebral artery compression (VAC). VAC can be done manually or by Doppler probe. The effects of VAC were evaluated with EEG and EOG.

Materials and Methods

Seven patients suffering from VBIPH were recorded in quantified EEG cartography. All the patients have been submitted to a complete investigation including neurological, ENT, CT scan, digital intra-arterial bihumeral angiography, and CBF examination by 133 Xe [3]. The EEG recordings were done by CARTOVAR, ALVAR. Before VAC, three recordings of 6 s each were analyzed and mapping was done on the average.

VAC has been carried out: (1) in the sitting position VAC of the left then the right artery by Doppler probe; (2) in standing position VAC of the left then the right vertebral artery always with Doppler probe.

The VAC lasted 6 s, during which EEG recordings and maps were done. The mapping variations were analyzed for each vertebral artery, for theta and delta, in sitting and standing positions (table I). A positive response was an increase in the power of delta or theta band during VAC. The results were expressed with data of 8 recordings (2 corresponding at delta and theta, 2 for each vertebral artery, 2 for each position).

For EOG, the technique was described elsewhere in detail [4]. Briefly, we analyzed the saccadic eye movements. A pseudo-random stimulus of 40° was used. Amplitude, accuracy and maximum velocities of saccades were computerized on-line by a minicomputer IN 110. VAC lasted 13 s.

Table I. Sex, age and abnormality for each patient

Patient	Sex	Age	VAC		EEG evaluation: position		Delta	Theta	Mapping	EOG: VAC	
			R	L	sitting	standing				R	L
Peg	M	51	2/4	4/4	3/4	3/4	2/4	4/4	asym. L	hypo. +	hyper. +
Vin	F	53	2/4	3/4	2/4	3/4	2/4	3/4	asym. R	hyper+ slow	hyper. ++
Iaf	F	54	4/4	1/4	3/4	2/4	2/4	3/4	sym.	hypo. +	hypo. +
Dess	M	58	0/4	1/4	1/4	0/4	1/4	0/4	sym.	–	hyper. +
Fev	F	58	–	2/4	1/2	1/2	0/2	2/4	asym. L	–	hyper. +
Now	F	67	1/4	1/4	1/4	1/4	1/4	1/4	asym. R	–	–
But	F	75	–	2/2	2/2	–	1/1	1/1	asym. R	–	hyper. slow +++

R = Right; L = left; asym. = asymmetric; sym. = symmetric; hypo. = hypometry; hyper. = hypermetry; slow = slowing of the maximum velocity.

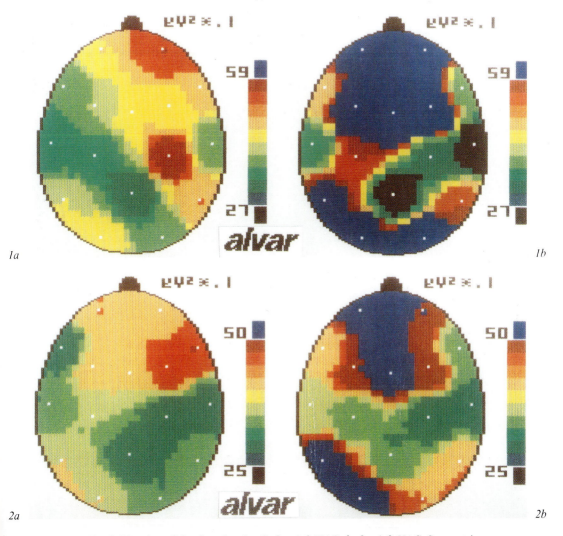

Fig. 1. Mapping of the theta band. *a* Before left VAC; *b* after left VAC. Symmetric increase in power in anterior and posterior regions.

Fig. 2. Mapping of the theta band. *a* Before left VAC; *b* after left VAC. Asymmetric increase in power in left Rolandic and parieto-occipital regions.

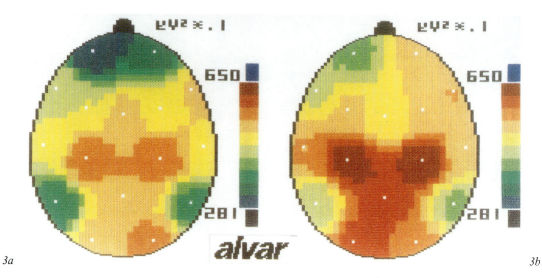

3a   *3b*

Fig. 3. Mapping of the delta band. *a* Before left VAC; *b* after left VAC. Symmetric increase in power in central regions.

Results

After VAC, 3 types of induced anomalies can be seen in EEG maps: (1) Symmetric increase in power of theta and/or delta bands in anterior (frontal) and/or posterior (occipito-parietal) regions (fig. 1). (2) Asymmetric increase in power of theta and/or delta bands in anterior and/or posterior regions (fig. 2). (3) Symmetric bilateral and central increase in power of theta and/or delta bands (fig. 3).

These increases were independent of the patient's position but were related to the VAC of the dominant vertebral artery and the severity of VBI. A positive response in 'delta' seems more representative of a long disabling VBI.

In EOG, we also found 3 types of induced anomalies after VAC: a hypermetry (without post-saccadic drift) or a hypometry of the saccade. In long and severe VBI, slowing of the saccade can be induced. All these anomalies are reversible in 8–15 min.

Discussion

Actually, in the hypothesis of a provoked ischemia in the posterior fossa an increase in power of delta and/or theta can be found. Symmetrical anterior and/or posterior increases of delta and theta power are found in intoxications or in cervical traumatisms when there is a vigilance perturbation. A brief increase of power in the delta band, spreading over the entire scalp, is roughly similar to NREM sleep.

EOG anomalies (hypermetria) have been described in cerebellar diseases, while hypometria is found in brain stem, cerebellum and basal ganglia diseases. Slowing of the saccades is typical of brain stem lesions, such as pontine reticular formation disturbances.

Conclusion

In VBIPH, quantified EEG cartography and computerized EOG are two noninvasive methods that can measure objectively the reproducible effects of VAC. These tests are useful to prove the diagnosis and to evaluate the severity of the VBI.

Acknowledgment

We are very indebted to Laboratoires SPECIA (France) for their financial support to this publication.

References

1   Ausmann, J.I.; Shrontz, C.E.; Pearce, J.E.; Diaz, F.G.; Cerelius, J.L.: Vertebrobasilar insufficiency. Archs Neurol. *42:* 803–808 (1985).
2   Barnett, H.J.M.: Progress towards stroke prevention. Robert Warturbery lecture. Neurology *11:* 1212–1225 (1980).
3   Rancurel, G.; Freyss, G.; Kieffer, E.; Vitte, E.; Luizy, F.; Raynaud, C.; Lassen, N.A.; Buge, A.: L'insuffisance vertébrobasilaire de type postural hémodynamique. Sem. Hôp. Paris *62:* 2741–2754 (1986).
4   Vitte, E.; Freyss, G.; Rancurel, G.; Raynaud, P.; Pialoux, P.; Zakki, A.: Eye tracking anomalies induced by vertebral artery compression in vertebrobasilar insufficiency. A computer assisted study. Correlations with results of other neurophysiological explorations. Bárány Soc. Meet., Ann Arbor 1985.

C. Sebban, MD, Hôpital Charles Foix, F-94200 Ivry (France)

Subject Index